TO RAISE UP THE MAN FARTHEST DOWN

TO RAISE UP THE MAN FARTHEST DOWN

TUSKEGEE UNIVERSITY'S
Advancements in Human Health,
1881–1987

DANA R. CHANDLER and EDITH POWELL

Foreword by LINDA KENNEY MILLER

The University of Alabama Press
Tuscaloosa

The University of Alabama Press
Tuscaloosa, Alabama 35487-0380
uapress.ua.edu

Inquiries about reproducing material from this work should be addressed to the
University of Alabama Press.

Typeface: Caslon and Scala Sans

Cover image: From top left, clockwise: Dr. Russell Brown checking cell cultures;
Jeanne M. Walton examining HeLa cells; Tuskegee's hospital nurses, c. 1920; all
courtesy of the Tuskegee University Archives.
Cover design: Michele Myatt Quinn

Library of Congress Cataloging-in-Publication Data

Names: Chandler, Dana R. (Dana Ray), 1958- author. | Powell, Edith, 1940-
author.
Title: To raise up the man farthest down : Tuskegee University's advancements
in human health, 1881–1987 / Dana R. Chandler and Edith Powell ; foreword by
Linda Kenney Miller.
Description: Tuscaloosa : The University of Alabama Press, [2018] | Includes
bibliographical references and index.
Identifiers: LCCN 2017053878| ISBN 9780817319892 (cloth) | ISBN 9780817391911
(ebook)
Subjects: | MESH: Tuskegee University. | Universities—history | Biomedical
Research—history | Health Services—history | Poliovirus Vaccines—history
| Race Relations—history | History, 19th Century | History, 20th Century |
Alabama
Classification: LCC R746.A2 | NLM W 19 AA4 | DDC 610.71/176149—dc23
LC record available at https://lccn.loc.gov/2017053878

Contents

Figures

Abbreviations and Acronyms

GWCRF	George Washington Carver Research Foundation (also, CRF for short)
HBCUs	Historically Black Colleges and Universities
JAAMH	John A. Andrew Memorial Hospital (also, JAH for short)
MOD	March of Dimes
NFIP	National Foundation for Infantile Paralysis
USPHS	US Public Health Service
USPHSSS	US Public Health Service Syphilis Study

Foreword

To Raise Up the Man Farthest Down: Tuskegee University's Advancements in Human Health, 1881–1987 provides a timely and important historical account of significant advances in health care made in Tuskegee over the span of more than a century. In this book, Dana R. Chandler and Edith Powell have meticulously researched and presented comprehensive evidence that supports their thesis that the contributions of five Tuskegee presidents resulted in extraordinary advances in quality health care that impacted millions of lives worldwide.

Under the leadership of Dr. Booker T. Washington, founding president of Tuskegee Institute (now University), John A. Andrew Memorial Hospital was built on the campus to provide medical care for students, faculty, staff, and residents in the surrounding rural areas. A School of Nursing was established, and the John A. Andrew Clinical Society was formed to bring physicians of all races from across the nation to Tuskegee each year to perform surgeries and provide free medical services to patients from the region and to provide postgraduate medical training for thousands of black doctors who were barred from white institutions. Washington believed that a healthy community is a viable community and established Health Improvement Week (later National Negro Health Week), which was observed annually for thirty-five years. The campaign for better health continued after Washington's death in 1915.

Robert Moton, Tuskegee's second president (1915–1935), collaborated with Dr. John A. Kenney, developer of John A. Andrew Memorial Hospital, along with the National Medical Association and the NAACP to ensure that the veterans hospital being funded and constructed by the US government at Tuskegee in 1923 would be staffed by black medical personnel. Moton was responsible for the only chapter of the Red Cross for black people in the world, and his relationship with philanthropist Julius Rosenwald led to the establishment of educational programs and opportunities for black children in the Tuskegee community and across the South.

Dr. Frederick D. Patterson, Tuskegee's third president (1935–1953), founded the School of Veterinary Medicine and the United Negro College Fund. Under his helm and with cooperation from the National Foundation for Infantile Paralysis, Tuskegee opened a unit for infantile paralysis treatment and research at the John A. Andrew Memorial Hospital in 1941. Under Patterson's tenure, Tuskegee's nursing program became the first accredited baccalaureate program in Alabama in 1948. Tuskegee continued to be the center of health care for black patients in Alabama and throughout the South.

Dr. Luther H. Foster, Tuskegee's fourth president (1953–1981), shepherded the institution through the tumultuous civil rights movement. He oversaw the establishment of the Occupational Therapy and Clinical Lab Science programs and the development of a strong Engineering Department. He encouraged students to intern at the VA Hospital to ensure marketability and employability. Tuskegee's Carver Research Foundation collaborated with the National Foundation for Infantile Paralysis in the development of Jonas Salk's polio vaccine, and their work with HeLa cells is now being widely recognized. HeLa cells are named after Henrietta Lacks and identified by the first two letters of her first and last names. Lacks died of cancer on October 4, 1951, and the line of her cervical cancer cells has proven to be so robust and productive that they have continued to be useful into the twenty-first century.

Dr. Benjamin F. Payton, Tuskegee's fifth president (1981–2010), followed in his predecessors' footsteps by establishing the Tuskegee University National Center for Bioethics in Research and Health Care as the result of President Bill Clinton's apology on behalf of the nation for the infamous Tuskegee Syphilis Study. In 1985, Tuskegee Institute started offering doctoral programs in science and engineering and was therefore elevated to university status. The scope of this book covers the events between the university's founding in 1881 through 1987, two years after this transition.

To Raise Up the Man Farthest Down recognizes the tenures of each of these Tuskegee presidents for their efforts to eradicate the racial, social, and cultural obstacles that they faced in their collective quest to maintain fidelity to the mission first espoused by Dr. Washington: high quality educational programs, effective public health policies, and equal opportunity. Progress made under each administration benefited the entire community and was integral to Tuskegee's success in enhancing the quality of life for all—including "the man farthest down."

Linda Kenney Miller, granddaughter of John A. Kenney, MD, and author of *Beacon on the Hill*

Acknowledgments

My heartfelt thanks must go to Elizabeth Gregory North for her review and suggestions and support of the manuscript; without her support I cannot write. Also, special thanks to Breanna Chandler Yarbrough for her skillful review and comments throughout the process, but especially to the final draft.

To the "Tuskegee Gang" who have put up with our sporadic meetings and discussions during these last four years while writing on this story: Jim McSwain, Glenn Drummond, Tim and Kelly Bryant, Keri Hallford, Shirley Curry, and Lanice Middleton. Thank you for your patience and friendship.

To my own special support group: Betty P. Fisher, Rebecca G. Veal, Elaine W. Helms, Teresa H. Chandler, and Dr. Marceline Egnin. Your willingness to listen and offer suggestions and criticisms when needed, as well as your support, always, provided the wind beneath my wings. You are a blessing.

To Cheryl Ferguson, assistant archivist: a special friend and outstanding resource. Thank you for your patience in searching for documents for me over the years of this writing. I am forever grateful.

To the University of Alabama Press, especially Elizabeth Motherwell, Senior Acquisitions Editor for the Natural Sciences, who has championed our story since the beginning; Blanche Sarratt, Marketing Coordinator; and Joanna Jacobs, Assistant Managing Editor. Thanks and gratitude for your belief in our story, for your advocacy and guidance during the editing process, and for your overall support throughout the entire publication process. Also, thanks to the outside readers (you know who you are); your comments made this a better story.

Finally, but not the least, to my colleague and friend Dana R. Chandler: my forever thanks for your patience, support, encouragement, and knowledge-sharing during these long but rewarding months of writing. This book certainly would not have happened without your brilliance at computer skills and

your historical writing genius. I learned very early in the preliminary discussions that the vocabulary of my medical background was not enough to enrich and qualify this story as a historical book. Without your understanding and willingness to listen to my thoughts expressed in medical vocabulary, then your help to re-form them into the accepted historical vernacular, the distinctive part of the story that I had to contribute would not have been as acceptable to the community of historical writers and publishers. What a great ride, laughs, at times some tension, much patience and untold hours of searching for the most exciting words and phrases; and, the absolute best outcome: Yes, we are still friends.
— Edith Powell

My acknowledgments must start with my coauthor and dear friend, Edith Powell. Edie, as her friends call her, is a special individual. She is both gentle and intense, brilliant and accommodating, and, above all, patient with someone who is demanding and precise in his writing. I am not a medical expert. In fact, I am a novice in every respect. Edie's intimate knowledge of medical terminology and techniques, particularly regarding polio treatment, made this work possible. Simply, it would not have been possible for me to write anything without her. Thank you, "my Edie."

My daughter, Breanna Chandler Yarbrough, has proven to be helpful to me time and again as an editor and advocate. Brilliant and accommodating, all I must do is ask and she readily spends her energy in doing whatever is needed. Thank you, Breanna for reading and rereading this work. Your comments and suggestions have directly contributed to its success.

To my friends and colleagues, also known as the "Tuskegee Gang," thank you. Jim McSwain, Glenn Drummond, Tim and Kelly Bryant, Keri Hallford, Shirley Curry, and Lanice Middleton have helped with their support, suggestions and patience during a long and arduous process. A special thanks to Jared McWilliams for scanning the images.

To my supervisor and friend Juanita Roberts, thank you for believing in me and supporting me in my work here at Tuskegee University. The opportunity to work here during your tenure as Director of Library Services has made my job pleasant and satisfying. This job made writing this book easier.

To Cheryl Ferguson, my colleague and friend, thank you for all that you have done to make this possible. You aided us with researching, by making suggestions, and by holding off interruptions. Again, thank you so much.

Thank you to the wonderful staff at the University of Alabama Press. You kept believing in us and pushing us.

To Tuskegee University and the people that preceded me, you are the reason for this book. Your legacy has provided the fodder for every page. God, in

His infinite wisdom, knew this is where I should be. I love this institution. Thank you.

Finally, to my wonderful wife and best friend, Teresa, you always know how to keep me grounded and you never let me forget where my priorities should be. Thank you for loving me and believing in me.

— Dana R. Chandler

Introduction

Overcoming the Challenges of Our Past

The investment in things that make for health, for prosperity, for upright living, those things immediately yield their profit to all who will encourage them.

—Booker T. Washington

Mention Tuskegee University[1] to just about anyone, and you will get the same reply: "Oh that's the home of Booker T. Washington and George Washington Carver." Sometimes, they may mistake it for the location of the infamous Tuskegee Syphilis Study or only associate it with the famous Tuskegee Airmen. While these are all important pieces of Tuskegee's history, the university is more than these. It is also home to the National Negro Business League and the National Negro Health Week.[2] It is the alma mater of the first black[3] woman to win a gold medal at an Olympics and to coach an Olympic team.[4] It is where the first four-star black general earned his undergraduate degree and where the principal protagonist in the pivotal 1961 Civil rights Supreme Court case *Gomillion v. Lightfoot* taught classes.[5] It is also the location of the laboratory used to mass-produce the cell cultures used in the field trials for the Salk and Sabin vaccines, allowing research that eventually led to an almost complete eradication of polio[6] in the United States. Historically, Tuskegee has been a leader among black colleges and universities, including sports, social issues, research, and health care. Although the university's involvement in sports and social issues has been highly touted and investigated, its work in research and health care has received little acknowledgement.

Tuskegee University has been intimately involved with health care since its inception, fulfilling Booker T. Washington's vision of healthy minds and bodies.[7] Unfortunately, many have the erroneous impression there is little more to learn about Tuskegee's role in science[8] and medicine. Its contributions have been overshadowed by the infamous US Public Health Service Syphilis Study. This so-called study was actually an ethical travesty: from 1932 to 1972, 600 black men in Macon County (399 of whom already had syphilis) were told they were being treated for a generalized ailment dubbed "bad blood" when in reality, none of the patients were given any treatment at all—even though the ef-

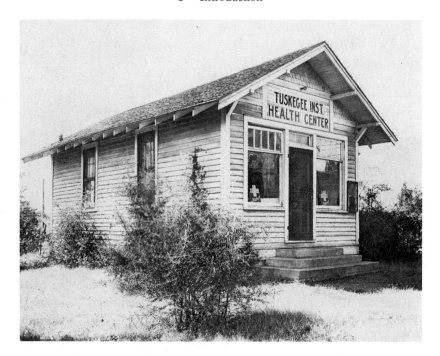

Figure 1. The original Tuskegee Institute infirmary, established by Booker T. Washington for the care of students. (Courtesy of the Tuskegee University Archives)

fects of untreated syphilis were already universally understood, and even after a cure for syphilis was widely available. After the study finally ended in the 1970s, it became a national outrage—a symbol for scientific racism that greatly increased public awareness of the issues of medical ethics and informed consent. Although the university did not itself instigate, run, or house the study, it was involved with the study's initial inception.

In 1929, the US Public Health Service, with funding from the Julius Rosenwald Fund, sponsored a syphilis treatment pilot program in five Southern states to determine the prevalence, and eventual treatment, of the disease among rural African American populations. Because it was initially characterized as a humanitarian effort, Tuskegee's then-president, Robert Moton, agreed to throw the institute's support behind it if "Tuskegee Institute [got] its full share of the credit" and some black medical professionals were given the opportunity to take part. Fortunately, Moton's request was not followed through with, and Tuskegee was able to avoid any future embarrassment for complicity in the latter, more infamous study. The initial Rosenwald-funded version of the study came to an end in 1932 when there was a lack of matching funds from local jurisdictions.[9] The federal government used the Rosenwald study findings to determine the location for their later work. The idea that that the so-called Tuskegee Syphlilis Study was initiated or administered by Tuskeege University is a misconception.

Conversely, Macon County (of which the town of Tuskegee is the county seat) was also the site of pioneering work by Tuskegee University researchers that supported the development of a preventative for infantile paralysis. It is no accident that some of the breakthrough work for the prevention of polio was conducted at Tuskegee. This came about because of a long history of efforts to advance scholarship, science, and technology beginning with the university's founders and continuing through its celebrated history. These were accomplished in spite of racism, scientific or otherwise.

Although Tuskegee excelled in promoting its graduates among the black community, especially during the 1940s, 1950s, and 1960s, the specter of racism hindered many in achieving their dreams and aspirations. Tuskegee became a haven for young intellectuals who came seeking knowledge in an environment that was singularly nurturing and nonoppressive. Unfortunately, after graduation, they were hindered not only by segregation, but also by a different type of racism.

Racism can be simply defined as a form of propaganda used to promote the superiority of one race over another, but it is also a social and political construct used to justify the bias and exploitation of a group that deems itself "superior" to a group deemed "inferior" for economic and political gains.[10] In fact, the concept of "race" is a rather new one, seeming to rise out of the ugly process of slavery.[11] Enslaved black people, who were often uneducated, having originated in or descended from a foreign culture with different customs and religions, were seen as incapable of meeting European standards of custom, religion, and culture.[12] Scientific racism,[13] which promotes the idea that one group of people is intellectually or physiologically superior to another, has its origins within the United States, specifically with Darwinist thought that propagated the notion that "primitive peoples could not be assimilated into a complex, white civilization."[14] Science has nothing to do with race or racism.[15]

The idea of scientific racism entered the mainstream during the latter half of the nineteenth century when men such as Arthur Gobineau, Vacher de Lapouge, and Johann Gottfried Herder sought to rank people based upon their supposed genetic origins within a specific region or nation.[16] Distinctions were made between the "civilized races," which were seen as having all the trappings of a "higher civilization," and the "savage races," which were seen as living only a notch above wild animals.[17] This led many to classify the "savages" as similar to animals, resulting in these people, like animals, having little to no rights. This situation was further exacerbated by political leaders who confirmed such views in their rhetoric.

Thomas Jefferson, the third president of the United States and author of the words "we hold these truths to be self-evident, that all men are created equal," also wrote, "I advance it, therefore, as a suspicion only, that the blacks . . . are inferior to the whites in the endowment of body and mind."[18] Several years later, while speaking at a debate, Abraham Lincoln, the sixteenth president of the United States, stated, "there is a physical difference between the white and black races, which I believe forbid the two races living together on terms of social and political equality."[19] Both of these men epitomized their time periods as leaders and thinkers, but their views on race were influenced by flawed methodologies and ideologies of men guided by their prejudices seeking to prove they were greater than others. Even though there were factions opposed to the institutions of slavery and racism, scientific racism was ingrained within much of American society from its inception onward.

Scientific racism did not decline with the coming of the new century. While Booker T. Washington and W. E. B. Du Bois were diligently working toward the betterment of black people through education, others were proclaiming the futility of such works. In his 1916 work, *The Psychology of the Negro*, George O. Ferguson wrote, "the Negro's intellectual deficiency is registered in the retardation percentages of the schools as well as in mental tests. And in view of all the evidence it does not seem possible to raise the scholastic attainment of the Negro to an equality with that of the white. It is probable that no expenditure of time or of money would accomplish this end, since education cannot create mental power, but can only develop that which is innate."[20]

This concept was reinforced with the works of Lewis Terman and others. Terman posited, "No amount of school instruction will ever make them intelligent voters or capable citizens."[21] This belief contributed to the then popular notion of eugenics, which is defined as "The science of racial purity and improvement . . . According to eugenic theory, people of different races inherited not only differences in appearance, moral character, and sexual behavior, but also differential susceptibility to disease. Doctors schooled in eugenic theory included these 'racial' distinctions as part of their diagnostic expectation, understanding disease susceptibility and medical outcomes differently for black and white patients."[22] Eugenics arose from the "social Darwinist" theory of the 1890s, leading to a myriad of tests and experimentations by some white scientists in an attempt to satisfy their notions of distinct physiological differences between the races.[23]

Men such Robert Bennet Bean, often considered one of the fathers of "scientific racism," and Raymond Vonderlehr and Taliaferro Clark, both of the US Public Health Service, subscribed to the notion of continued testing on black patients to confirm such things as the "alarming susceptibility to tuberculosis and venereal diseases."[24] Finally, Tulane University professor William

Benjamin Smith wrote: "If [black people] were the highest form of human life, we might be concerned . . . [but] to the clear, cold eye of science, the plight of these backward peoples appears practically hopeless. They have neither part nor parcel in the future history of man."[25] Yet, to the contrary, black people had been making significant contributions to the nation and society from its foundation.

Men such as Benjamin Banneker (1731–1806)—a self-taught astronomer and author who published an almanac containing information on eclipses, tide tables, and medicinal formulas—were the antithesis of the false conception of black people being incapable of intellectual accomplishments. Known for aiding in the establishment of the boundaries of Washington, DC, Banneker would eventually send Thomas Jefferson a copy of his first almanac in response to Jefferson's claims about black inferiority.[26] Others, such as Dr. Daniel Hale Williams (1858–1931), who in 1893 performed the first operation on the human heart, and Garret A. Morgan (1877–1963), who in 1923 invented the traffic signaling system, have remained rather anonymous in history, although their contributions were significant.[27] Women also made noteworthy contributions. Sarah E. Goode (1850–1905) was the first black woman in the United States to receive a patent (on July 14, 1885) for her invention of the cabinet bed,[28] and Madame C. J. Walker (1867–1919) is well known for developing a conditioning system for straightening hair.[29] Many others have contributed to the welfare of Americans and the world, yet continue to remain unknown and forgotten. As Du Bois stated, "silence and neglect of science can let truth utterly disappear or be unconsciously distorted."[30] Fortunately, while the aforementioned still experienced scientific racism, they were not hindered in their endeavors by their proposed lack of intellectual ability.

Although much was published about the differences between the "races," by the middle of the twentieth century, scientific racism as a theory began to retreat. Egalitarian ideas developed among a variety of scientific, political, and sociological ideologies that questioned "the notion of fixed and stable racial types."[31] Research has shown "the changing demography of the sciences, the increase in female and minority members in their ranks, had a definite impact on theoretical perspectives and methods."[32] By the late 1940s, the horrors of Nazi racism, and particularly anti-Semitism, drew into sharp contrast the problems faced by black people within the United States. This coupled with the internment of Japanese and German Americans during the war further pushed the international community to focus on the dissonance between American ideology, such as democracy and equality, and racial segregation. Finally, the information collected and assimilated by researchers that espoused the concept of scientific racism were soon shown to have had skewed results and faulty analysis.[33] By the mid- to late 1950s, scientific racism as a viable tenant of human classification had begun to wane, yet segregation in the United States was still going strong.

During the modern American civil rights movement, racism was confronted on every front. Late in the 1960s, civil rights icon Stokely Carmichael coined a phrase that defined much of the racism found within science: "institutional racism." The term was used to designate racial discrimination and segregation by powerful and influential religious or secular organizations.[34] Although institutional racism and scientific racism appear to be the same, the subtle dissimilarity comes not with physiological differences but with control and the arrogance of a supposed intellectual and academic superiority. Maulana Karenga argued that the effects of something like institutional racism "involved redefining African humanity to the world, poisoning past, present, and future relations with others who only know us through this stereotyping and thus damaging the truly human relations among peoples."[35] This definition aptly describes the situation many young African American scientists faced when it came to employment in health care and medical-related fields.

This became the work of Tuskegee University: overcoming the past that included racial stereotypes and prejudices to promote its students to a brighter future, on equal footing with all of mankind. The title of our book is itself a term drawn from the work of the esteemed Booker T. Washington, who—like so many of the university's finest—fought to raise up Tuskegee's students and all of black America. Such a lofty goal could only be accomplished through the diligent work of its presidents, administration, faculty, and staff who amply provided students with knowledge and confidence to be professionally competitive with any other graduates of higher learning institutions anywhere in the world.

I

Tuskegee's Commitment to Health Care

An Overview

I am exceedingly anxious that every young man and woman should keep a
hopeful and cheerful spirit as to the future. Despite all of our disadvantages
and hardships, ever since our forefathers set foot upon the American soil
as slaves our pathway has been marked by progress . . . I believe that we are
going to reach our highest development largely along the lines of scientific
and industrial education.

—Booker T. Washington

Tuskegee University developed through the efforts of Lewis Adams, a former
slave, and George W. Campbell, a former slave owner, who saw in the late 1870s
a need for the education of black residents of rural Macon County, Alabama.[1]
The founding date of the university was July 4, 1881, authorized by House Bill
165 of the Alabama Legislature. Tuskegee's history is closely linked to the accomplishments of its presidents who continued to be the driving force behind
the educational, sociological, and health care advances at the school.

From a modest beginning in a one-room shanty located near Butler's Chapel
AME Zion Church, Tuskegee University rose to national prominence under
the leadership of its first president, Booker T. Washington.[2] Washington (figure 3) was a highly skilled organizer and fund-raiser who counseled US presidents and was a strong advocate of black farmers and businesses. He worked
tirelessly in developing methods to aid black people to succeed by establishing
a variety of on-campus vocational classes including carpentry, brick-making,
sewing, millinery, animal husbandry, and gardening.

Students were also required to complete coursework toward general diplo-
mas, which included mathematics, English, and history. Student enrollment
was not limited to rural Macon County and the South but was international in
composition. Furthermore, Washington's vision for Tuskegee University (originally called Tuskegee Normal and changed to Tuskegee Normal and Industrial
Institute in 1893) involved recruiting the best and brightest available within
the black community, including George Washington Carver (1860–1943), who
came to Tuskegee as farm manager in 1896; architect Robert R. Taylor (1868–
1942), who started as director of Mechanical Industries in 1882; and Monroe N.

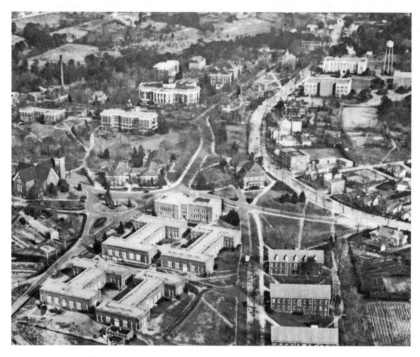

Figure 2. Aerial view of Tuskegee University, c. 1940. (Courtesy of the Tuskegee University Archives)

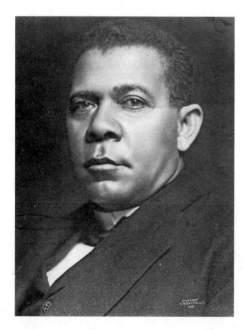

Figure 3. Booker T. Washington, Tuskegee's first president. (Courtesy of the Tuskegee University Archives)

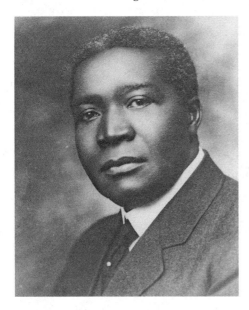

Figure 4. Robert Moton. (Courtesy of the Tuskegee University Archives)

Work (1866–1945), who was founder of the Department of Records and Research (later called the archives).[3]

Washington's emphasis on health care at Tuskegee began almost immediately. Students who came to Tuskegee were raised on staples such as turnip greens, salt pork, and cornbread.[4] Many students were unhealthy and incapable of meeting the rigors of work required during their time at Tuskegee. Aware that the health of his students required more than a change in diet, Washington sought to help their families through education. By helping the families, he could help the students.[5] From the Jesup Wagon to the National Negro Health Week, he utilized a variety of methods to reach the poor in an attempt to provide a more healthful environment for them and their families. In 1913, he started an on-site clinic to provide medical treatment to students, faculty, and staff, which later developed into the John A. Andrew Memorial Hospital.

Tuskegee University's prominence as a black school of education and industrial training[6] did not end after the untimely death of Washington in 1915. Under the tenure of Robert Moton, Tuskegee's second president, the university continued to grow in size and prestige. Moton (figure 4) actively solicited for more adequate buildings and modern equipment for teaching the trades, more comfortable housing for faculty and students, and enlarged and improved facilities for recreation, health, and academic studies. In 1927, Moton raised the university's academic program from high school level to full four-year college status, with bachelor degrees available in agriculture, home economics, mechanical industries, and education. Furthermore, through his efforts, the

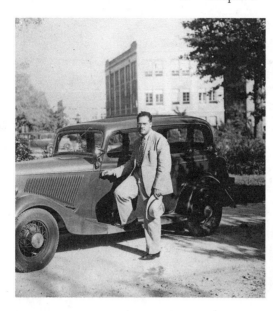

Figure 5. Frederick D. Patterson. (Courtesy of the Tuskegee University Archives)

university donated land for the Tuskegee Veterans Administration Hospital (1923),[7] the first hospital in the United States staffed entirely by black professionals. Like his predecessor, Moton was an accomplished fund-raiser and recruiter. He continued the institutional relationship with financiers such as Julius Rosenwald (1862–1932) begun by Washington, which led to the establishment of a specific foundation to fund programs for underprivileged portions of society and the education of black people.

Moton's work with health care went beyond Tuskegee, especially as chairman of the Colored Advisory Commission during the 1927 Mississippi River Flood. Charged by Secretary of Commerce Herbert Hoover to help with problems encountered by African Americans affected by the destruction of levees adjacent to the Mississippi River, Moton worked to develop measures to provide displaced families adequate food, medical aid, and housing.

Tuskegee University's accomplishments continued with its third president, Dr. Frederick D. Patterson. As president, Patterson (figure 5) founded the School of Veterinary Medicine at Tuskegee in 1944 (in 2016, nearly 75 percent of all black veterinarians in America were Tuskegee graduates), the year he also founded the United Negro College Fund (UNCF). The UNCF continues today as a critical source of annual income for a consortium of Historically Black Colleges and Universities (HBCUs), including Tuskegee University.

During the 1940s, while the rest of the world was embroiled in war, the university continued to lead the way in working toward better health care for black patients nationwide. The Infantile Paralysis Center opened on January 15, 1941, as another unit of Tuskegee University's John A. Andrew Memorial Hospital (JAAMH). The center provided treatment facilities and services for black polio patients from the southeastern states, as well as care for Alabama patients with other orthopedic conditions. In 1948, the nursing program at Tuskegee University became the first baccalaureate program in the state of Alabama.

Further accomplishments came with the university's participation in the Civilian Pilot Training Program (which began at Tuskegee in 1939), eventually leading to the formation of the 99th Fighter Squadron of Tuskegee Airmen in June 1941. The men and women of this group represented some of the most courageous in the country. Not only were they fighting an enemy on foreign soil, but also they were fighting segregation and Jim Crow laws at home.

The fourth president, Dr. Luther H. Foster (figure 6), led Tuskegee through the turbulent years of the modern American civil rights movement, in addition to overseeing the organization of the College of Arts and Sciences, the elimination of several vocational programs, and the development of engineering programs. Under Foster's leadership, the University maintained an attitude of open dialogue, allowing a variety of speakers such as Martin Luther King Jr., Malcolm X, Stokely Carmichael, Julian Bond, and Alex Haley to visit campus.

Furthermore, faculty and staff were not discouraged from participating in the civil rights movement. Dr. Charles Gomillion (1900–1995), professor of Sociology and Dean of the College of Arts and Sciences, filed a lawsuit protesting the gerrymandering of Tuskegee's black citizens out of their right to vote, leading in 1960 to the groundbreaking Supreme Court case *Gomillion v. Lightfoot*. Tragically, on January 3, 1966, Tuskegee University freshman Samuel Younge Jr. (1944–1966) became the first currently enrolled black college student killed as a result of involvement in the civil rights movement.

In the late 1970s, Foster spearheaded the development of the Occupational Therapy and Clinical Laboratory Sciences programs (also known as Allied Health). The Occupational Therapy Program graduated its first class in 1980, making it the second-oldest such professional program in Alabama. The Clinical Laboratory Sciences Program was initiated in 1978 and later accredited in 1980.[8] Students participated in internships at the local veterans hospital, making them more marketable upon graduation.

Under the leadership of Tuskegee's fifth president, Dr. Benjamin F. Payton, the Tuskegee University National Center for Bioethics in Research and Health Care was founded in 1999[9] as a result of Payton's position on the Tuskegee Syphilis Study Legacy Committee. The legacy committee pursued a government apology for its participation in the US Public Health Service Syphilis Study, which had been conducted in Macon County, Alabama, from 1932 to

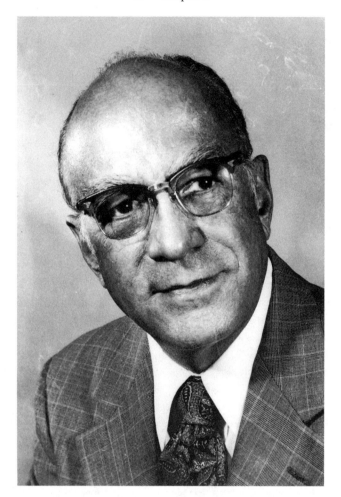

Figure 6. Luther H. Foster. (Courtesy of the Tuskegee University Archives)

1972. As a point of clarification, Tuskegee University did not as a whole participate in the study, which is contrary to what many in the media have insinuated.[10]

Payton's commitment to education was exemplified when, in 1985, Tuskegee attained university status and began offering its first doctoral programs in materials science and engineering. Unfortunately, due to a lack of a consistent revenue and support, Payton (figure 7) also was faced with the decision to close JAAMH in 1987. This meant nursing students and other students in the medical professions had to seek internships and employment at hospitals in other cities.

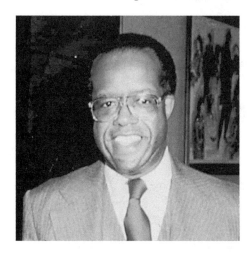

Figure 7: Benjamin F. Payton.
(Courtesy of the Tuskegee University Archives)

Tuskegee and Health Care, the Early Years

Tuskegee, though not a medical school, was heavily involved in providing its students, faculty, and staff adequate health care.[11] Booker T. Washington's philosophy of a healthy "head, hand and heart"[12] permeated every aspect of the school's teaching and training. Daily calisthenics and classes in hygiene were mandatory, beginning as early as 1881.[13] By the late 1880s, an infirmary was established in order to provide simple medical care for the sick. In 1901, a need for better treatment and health care led to the development of a hospital on campus. These events proved pivotal in Washington's continued evolution as an early leader in health care in the South.

By the end of his first decade at Tuskegee, Washington had already used his influence to recruit the first licensed black physician in the state of Alabama. Dr. Cornelius N. Dorsette, one of Washington's classmates at Hampton, started practicing as early as 1883.[14] Prior to his coming, most physicians in Alabama were unlicensed and, often, not academically trained.[15] In an article titled "The Negro Doctor in the South," published in the *Independent*, Washington noted: "When I went to Alabama in 1881, there was not a negro doctor, dentist or pharmacist in the State."[16] By 1907, there were "more than one-hundred Negro Doctors in the State of Alabama and there are over twenty-five in the Birmingham district."[17] Within fifteen years, Alabama had acquired black doctors in many of its major metropolitan areas. Unfortunately, this was still short of the numbers needed to adequately support the majority of the population.[18]

Dorsette (1852–1897), like Washington, was born during slavery, yet he became the second black graduate of the University of Buffalo medical school in 1882. Following graduation, he worked in various medical positions in New

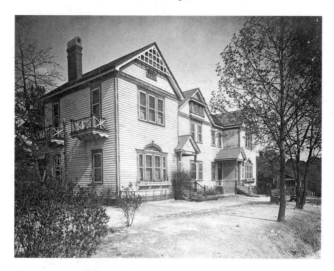

Figure 8. Pinecrest Hospital, Tuskegee University Campus.
(Courtesy of the Tuskegee University Archives)

York. Energetic and resourceful, Dorsette maintained a general practice while
working at the psychiatric ward of the hospital in Lyons, New York. He also
gained valuable experience working at the poor house and insane asylum of
Wayne County. At the behest of Washington, Dorsette visited Montgomery,
Alabama, and was determined to begin practicing medicine as soon as was
legally possible. In early 1883, he sat through a grueling six-day examination,
which was administered solely by white male physicians, in order to become
licensed to practice medicine in Alabama. He then became Washington's personal physician, a position Dorsette maintained until his death in 1897.[19]

Dorsette's legacy is further confirmed by his work in helping to establish
the first hospital for black patients in the state of Alabama. The hospital, located in Tuskegee, was called the Tuskegee Institute Hospital and Nurse Training School, and was opened in 1892 specifically "to provide care for the school's
faculty and students and to train black nurses."[20] One of the first physicians at
this newly created hospital was Halle Tanner Dillon (1865–1901), the first licensed female physician within the state of Alabama, who was mentored by
Dorsette.[21]

Dillon, born to a prominent African Methodist Episcopal (AME) Church
minister, Benjamin Tanner, graduated with honors from the Woman's Medical College of Pennsylvania. She had previously written to Booker T. Washington inquiring about a position at Tuskegee. Washington accepted Dillon
for the position of resident physician, contingent upon her passing the Alabama certification exam, the same exam that Dorsette had passed. Washington
arranged for Dillon to be tutored by Dorsette, and she passed the exam and

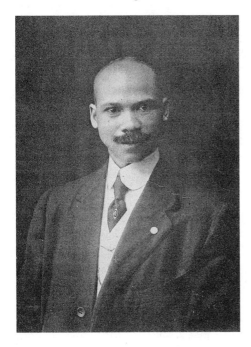

Figure 9. John A. Kenney, MD
(Courtesy of the Tuskegee University Archives)

began serving at Tuskegee on September 1, 1891. Interestingly, a white woman, Anna M. Longshore, had previously taken the exam but failed, leaving Dillon not only the first licensed black female physician, but also the first licensed female physician of any race in the state of Alabama. Dillon practiced at Tuskegee until sometime in 1894, when she married Tuskegee math teacher John Quincy Johnson, and they moved to Columbia, South Carolina, where he became president of Allen University. She died of dysentery on April 26, 1901, at the age of 37.[22]

Washington's vision and vigor resulted in numerous medical firsts both in Alabama and the nation. Washington knew his students at the institute would learn better if they were healthy, so he established an infirmary to provide care for those who were sick. Black patients had little to no access to clinics, hospitals, or county health departments within the state of Alabama.[23] It was Washington, not Dorsette nor Dillon, who, in January 1891, opened an infirmary located in the girl's dormitory. It was that infirmary that would later be expanded to become the Tuskegee Institute Hospital and Nurse Training School. In 1901, a Mrs. Bennet of New Haven, Connecticut, donated the funds to build a thirty-five bed, two-story hospital. Pinecrest (figure 8) opened the following year with a staff consisting of a "resident physician, a graduate and assistant head nurse, and about twenty student nurses-in-training."[24] The resident physician was Dr. John A. Kenney (1874–1950) (figure 9),[25] an energetic young man with a résumé comparable to his position.

John A. Kenney was born June 11, 1874, to ex-slaves John and Caroline Kenney in Albemarle County, Virginia.[26] Kenney graduated first in his class from Hampton University in Virginia in 1897 and received his medical degree from the Leonard Medical School of Shaw University in Raleigh, North Carolina, in 1901. Kenney interned at Freedman's Hospital in Washington, DC, and came to Tuskegee in 1902, where he was placed in charge of the institute's small hospital. Kenney also served as personal physician to both Booker T. Washington and George Washington Carver. From 1902 to 1922, he served as the director and surgeon-in-chief of the hospital and School of Nurses. The hospital would undergo major changes during his tenure as physician.[27]

Within a few short years, Pinecrest Hospital outgrew its space. In 1911, another generous donation totalling $55,000 was made by Elizabeth A. Mason.[28] This important donation was for the erection, furnishing, and modernization of the hospital and nurses' training school. Construction of the new facility was accomplished under the direction of African American architect Robert R. Taylor (1868–1942).[29] On February 21, 1913, the hospital, located on Tuskegee University property, was named John A. Andrew Memorial Hospital (figure 10) in memory of Mrs. Mason's grandfather, John Albion Andrew, the governor of Massachusetts from 1861–1866 and a staunch abolitionist. On Saturday, March 8, 1913, in honor of the opening of the hospital, the *Tuskegee Student*[30] printed an article emphasizing the regional importance of the facility and describing the students' contributions to the project: "for the colored people of the South, who have few or no hospitals of their own, and who are, as a rule, excluded from first-class treatment in the hospitals of the South. The John A. Andrew Memorial Hospital, which will be under the immediate direction of Dr. John A. Kenney, medical director of the institute, and president of the national medical association. . . . it is an imposing structure, fitted with every convenience known to hospital surgery . . . the building is largely the result of students' work—from the digging of the clay, the making and laying of the bricks, to the installation of the electrical work, the plumbing and steamfitting."[31] Mrs. Mason further supported her grandfather's ideals by helping black students obtain an education in medicine. One such student, Hildrus A. Poindexter (1901–1987),[32] attended Harvard Medical School and after graduation became the new hospital's first intern. Poindexter noted that he "found Tuskegee Institute made to order for a practical internship with research possibilities in epidemiology and preventive medicine."[33] This was a profound statement, considering Tuskegee's location and its isolation from major cities containing larger hospitals that offered a wider range of specialized medical care.

Washington put into motion the development of a conduit for training medical staff without starting a new school. Black medical schools did exist, but they did not have an adequate number of hospitals for doctors to perform their

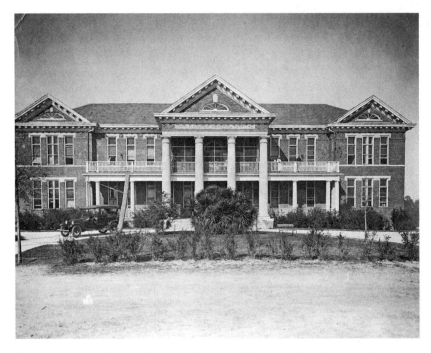

Figure 10. John A. Andrew Memorial Hospital. (Courtesy of the Tuskegee University Archives)

residencies. Besides, most medical schools and hospitals for black students and patients were located far to the north of Tuskegee, Alabama.

By 1860, there were nine medical schools, located specifically in northern states, which had admitted at least one black student for training.[34] Between 1860 and the early twentieth century, "the training of blacks in the field of medicine was discouraged in most cases unless the would-be doctor intended to practice in Liberia or some other country."[35] Prior to 1900, there were only two southern schools that granted medical degrees to black students: Howard University[36] and Meharry Medical College.[37] After the turn of the twentieth century, there were at least six additional medical schools, including the Flint Medical College of New Orleans and the Medical School of Shaw University in Raleigh, North Carolina. Five of those schools, not including Chattanooga Medical School (which closed in 1904) were closed after a report (compiled by Abraham Flexner for the Carnegie Foundation for the Advancement of Teaching)[38] noted that their programs were ineffectual and substandard. Only Howard and Meharry, which received grade-A accreditations, continued, providing the bulk of the country's black physicians from that point onward.[39]

John A. Andrew Memorial Hospital played an increasingly important role

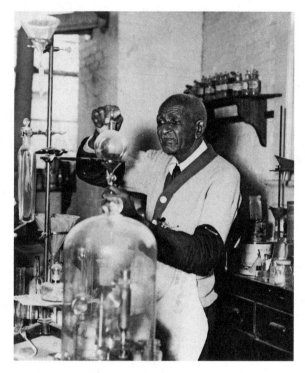

Figure 11. George Washington Carver in his laboratory.
(Courtesy of the Tuskegee University Archives)

in providing opportunities for both internships and residencies, thus fulfilling Washington's goal for providing Tuskegee students and graduates access to a top-tiered medical facility, staffed by some of the best doctors in the country. This reality met part of Washington's philosophy of a healthy "head, hand and heart," yet something else needed to be addressed.

Beyond the need for adequate ambulatory health care, Washington saw the poor health conditions of rural Southerners[40] and knew the causes—inadequate diet, bad eating habits, and lack of satisfactory sanitation—could be eliminated through education. Washington needed help, and in 1896, he brought in George Washington Carver (1864–1943) as director of the Tuskegee farm. Carver (figure 11) was instrumental in weaning "the Negro farmer (in Macon County-authors) away from the debilitating diet of meat, meal and molasses."[41] These ideas, and the programs developed through them, not only increased the overall health of the surrounding community, but also laid the foundation for one of the most important programs to come out of Washington's plan for comprehensive medical care: The John A. Andrew Clinic. This Clinic was instrumental in providing health care to the community, while also providing important training and continuing education for health-care professionals.

The John A. Andrew Clinic

The John A. Andrew Clinic (also called "the Clinic") was the catalyst that led to an influx of young black physicians who, due to a paucity of other approved sites, could come to Tuskegee to receive adequate experience in order to qualify to take their national board certifications.[42] The Clinic, which grew out of the efforts of many people including those affiliated with the National Medical Association (NMA), allowed interns or residents the opportunity to practice medicine, supervised by qualified doctors, on a wide variety of patients with a diversity of ailments.[43]

At a meeting of visiting physicians held in April 1912 at Tuskegee University, the first Clinic was inaugurated. During the first six years, attendees met without "any definite clinical organization,"[44] simply meaning they met without any formalized structure. Due to a rapid increase in membership, however, attendees at the meeting of April 4–6, 1917, voted to formalize the organization, naming it the John A. Andrew Clinical Society.

The Clinic, held each April in the John A. Andrew Memorial Hospital, provided a professional association between white and black physicians, during which new treatments were explained and medical experiences were exchanged. It is important to remember this was occurring at a period of time when black physicians were not allowed to practice at "white hospitals," nor were they allowed to participate in the white's only American Medical Association (AMA).[45] The Clinic, one of the foremost in the country, brought together leading figures from all branches of medicine.[46] It afforded the single opportunity many black physicians had in the southern region to meet with white colleagues for stimulation and growth.[47] They came from private and public practice, research facilities, and medical colleges, from both the north and the south, to exchange ideas, to report new methods, to ask questions, to explain techniques, and to participate in scholarly arguments. Disease, as they were aware, was not a black or white problem, but a human problem. The ideals the Clinic exemplified were the climax of the vision of Booker T. Washington, who understood medicine as the complex blending of the sciences of education, economics, health, and agriculture.[48] It is this vision he passed along to his students.[49]

The agenda for the weeklong Clinic (figure 12) consisted of lectures and paper presentations[50] by visiting specialists. Additionally, patient examinations during the Clinic provided "instruction for as many as 1,000 Negro physi-

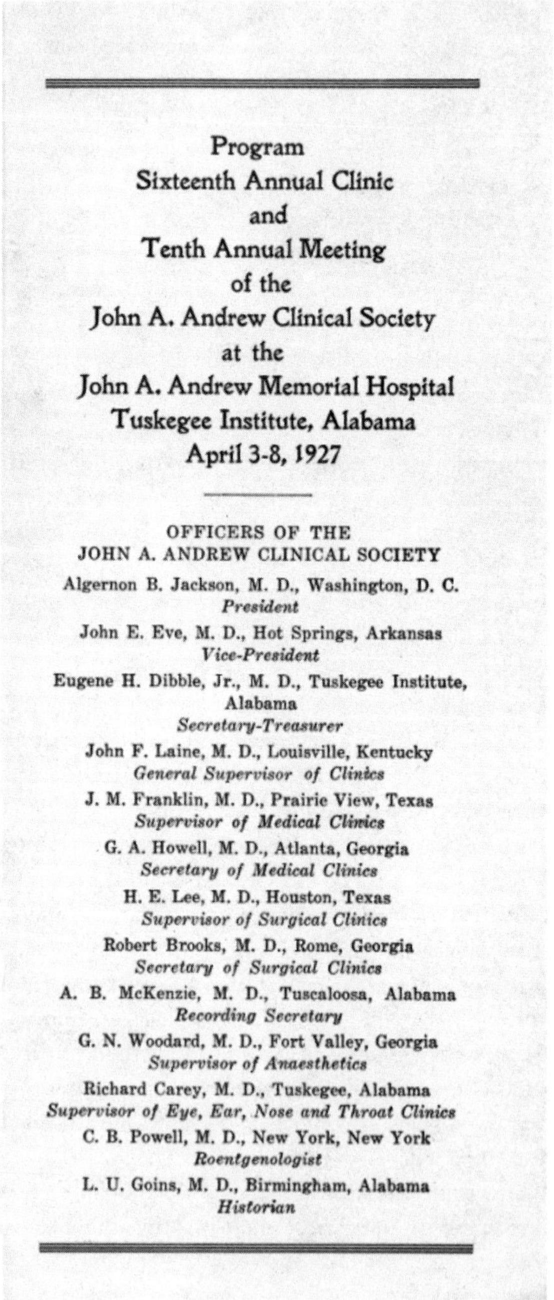

Program
Sixteenth Annual Clinic
and
Tenth Annual Meeting
of the
John A. Andrew Clinical Society
at the
John A. Andrew Memorial Hospital
Tuskegee Institute, Alabama
April 3-8, 1927

OFFICERS OF THE
JOHN A. ANDREW CLINICAL SOCIETY

Algernon B. Jackson, M. D., Washington, D. C.
President

John E. Eve, M. D., Hot Springs, Arkansas
Vice-President

Eugene H. Dibble, Jr., M. D., Tuskegee Institute,
Alabama
Secretary-Treasurer

John F. Laine, M. D., Louisville, Kentucky
General Supervisor of Clinics

J. M. Franklin, M. D., Prairie View, Texas
Supervisor of Medical Clinics

G. A. Howell, M. D., Atlanta, Georgia
Secretary of Medical Clinics

H. E. Lee, M. D., Houston, Texas
Supervisor of Surgical Clinics

Robert Brooks, M. D., Rome, Georgia
Secretary of Surgical Clinics

A. B. McKenzie, M. D., Tuscaloosa, Alabama
Recording Secretary

G. N. Woodard, M. D., Fort Valley, Georgia
Supervisor of Anaesthetics

Richard Carey, M. D., Tuskegee, Alabama
Supervisor of Eye, Ear, Nose and Throat Clinics

C. B. Powell, M. D., New York, New York
Roentgenologist

L. U. Goins, M. D., Birmingham, Alabama
Historian

Figure 12. Program of John A. Andrew Clinical Society,
1927. (Courtesy of the Tuskegee University Archives)

cians."[51] Areas within the hospital were set up according to medical specialties, each supervised by visiting specialists. Patients were seen and treated, with explanations, treatment protocols, techniques, and expected outcomes discussed between physicians, being referred elsewhere as necessary. Free treatment, including major surgical operations, was given yearly to more than 1,200 patients in the Tuskegee area.[52]

The visiting specialists were housed on the university campus, specifically at Dorothy Hall, and in local homes. Initially, the registration fee for the Clinic was $5.00, which did not include room and board.[53] Over the years, some of the specialists included Dr. Charles R. Drew, then head of the department of surgery at Howard University;[54] Dr. Reuben Kahn, University of Michigan, who developed the Kahn blood test for syphilis; Dr. Tinsley Harrison, dean of the University of Alabama Medical School (later named University of Alabama at Birmingham or UAB Medical School); and Dr. John Gorrell, director of medical services of the National Foundation for Infantile Paralysis.[55] The Clinic's rise in prestige prompted one newspaper to write: "the John A. Andrew Clinic, and the society that grew out of it, were to Negro health what Tuskegee Institute was to Negro education—symbols of rapid progress."[56]

The Clinic expanded to include programs for the participant's wives and other visitors.[57] Later, they added technical exhibits from a variety of major national suppliers such as Eli Lilly and Company, Parke-Davis and Company, Charles Pfizer and Company, and Wyeth, Inc.[58] They also included documentaries on a variety of medical and surgical procedures and diagnostic protocols, which were made available from the library of the AMA. These films were supplemental to the ongoing lectures and demonstrations.[59]

Washington and the National Negro Health Week

Robert Moton, the second president of Tuskegee University, wrote that the National Negro Health Week (NNHW) met Washington's philosophy of "*head, heart, hand,—and health.*"[60] Moton, who was the guiding force after Washington, further noted: "*It is an annual observance in which local, county, state, and national organizations of both races, as well as the Federal Government, now cooperate.*"[61]

In 1914, Washington viewed the poor health status of black Americans as an obstacle to economic progress and issued a call for "the Negro people . . . to join in a movement which shall be known as Health Improvement Week."[62] This eventually evolved into the National Negro Health Week, which would be observed annually for thirty-five years.

The NNHW (figure 13) was established in 1915 by Booker T. Washington. This was the last nationally organized effort made by Washington. Beginning

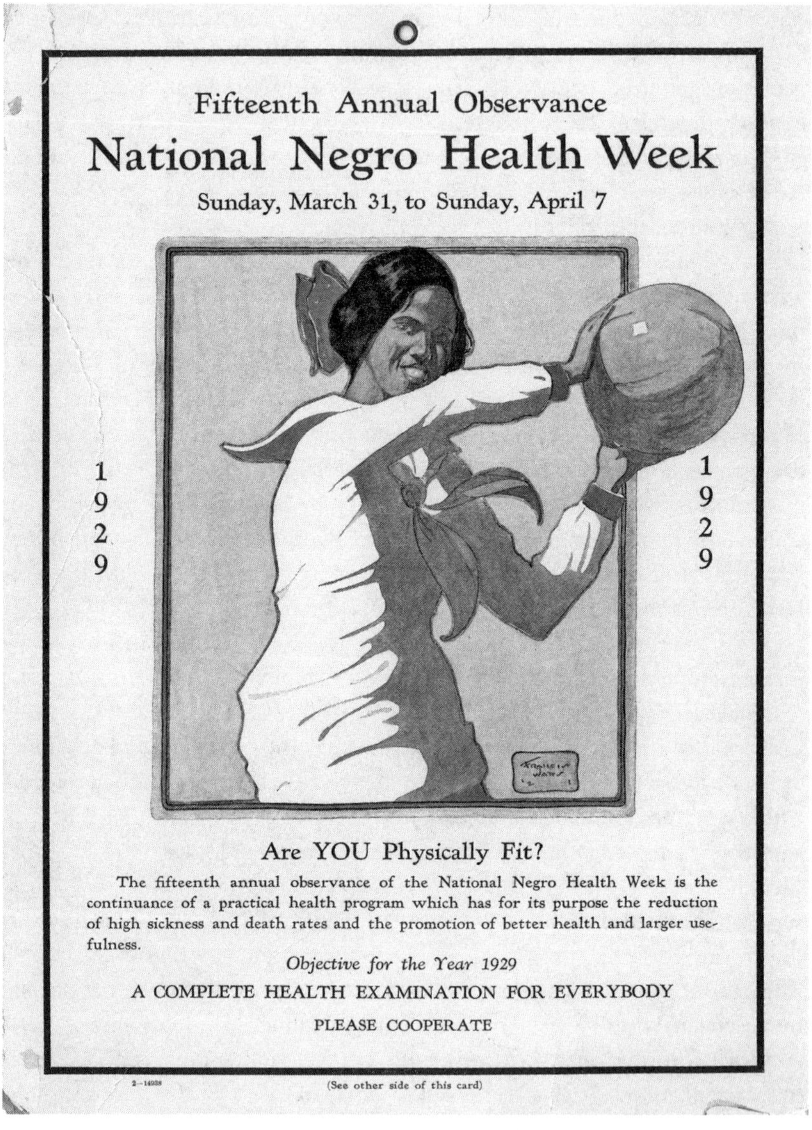

Figure 13. National Negro Health Week poster, 1929. (Courtesy of the Tuskegee University Archives)

in 1909, with sessions devoted to health at the Annual Tuskegee Negro Conference, the issue of health increasingly became an important aspect of this conference. As a result, a report was developed for the 1914 meeting concerning statistics that showed a higher mortality rate among African Americans. Suggestions were made in the report for methods to reduce the figures. The issue received nationwide attention, and Washington called for a Health Improvement Week for African Americans beginning the week of April 11, 1915. Working through several groups and organizations—which included teachers, ministers, and farmers' organizations—health officials were able to disseminate health information to African Americans. By 1930, the efforts of those involved with the program contributed to a rise in the average life span for African Americans from thirty-five to forty-five years.[63]

NNHW was the occasion for numerous activities associated with health issues. Programs during the week included lectures by health officials at schools, churches, and civic organizations with the aim of reaching the widest number of people. Officials were particularly interested in dealing with the health problems of children. Lectures for parents and children were organized, advertisements contracted, and children registered with local clinics. Doctors took advantage of the opportunity to promote their private practices. The majority of events related to local communities and circumstances.[64]

In many places, instead of holding health clinics in one place, the doctors and staff would travel around the communities. Leadership of the NNHW went through several changes that revealed the conflicts among leaders over bringing black people into the mainstream of American society. After Booker T. Washington's death in 1915, Robert Moton and educators from Tuskegee and other institutions were important in overseeing NNHW.

By the late 1920s, African American doctors associated with the NMA were instrumental in the planning and organization of the program. Physicians at Howard University Medical School headed the Planning Committee from 1930 to 1932, when Dr. Roscoe C. Brown,[65] a specialist in health education, became the director of the Office of Negro Health Work with the US Public Health Service (USPHS). Brown was also the only public health official to serve on President Franklin D. Roosevelt's "Black Cabinet." He would serve as director until the campaign was dissolved in 1950. Monroe N. Work served as secretary of the Planning Committee. Brown and Work were both employed by Tuskegee Institute at various times in their careers.

In 1930, the USPHS, with the help of the Julius Rosenwald Fund, took over organization of NNHW and expanded the concept to a year-round effort under the title "National Negro Health Movement."[66] By 1938, a new call was made to expand the number of agencies involved with NNHW. The majority of these new agencies, such as the American Heart Association, were for citizens of all races.

By World War II some national African American leaders argued for the end of annual NNHW campaigns in favor of the integration of African Americans into all aspects of society, including the health-care sector. This issue became known as the medical civil rights movement, which coincided with other civil rights issues of the 1940s. These leaders argued that all people should equally share all medical institutions and health programs. In 1950, the USPHS announced the end of the National Negro Health Movement on the grounds that the nation was moving toward integration. Some, like Louis T. Wright, a leader in the National Association for the Advancement of Colored People (NAACP), argued that separate black programs should not be accepted, even for humanitarian reasons. This goal, of course, had been on Washington's agenda all along.

Washington and the Jesup Wagon

During Washington's tenure, one of his greatest accomplishments in health care was the development of the Jesup Wagon and its associated programs.

Thomas Monroe (T. M.) Campbell, the first US Department of Agriculture Extension agent,[67] wrote: "Picture if you can the plight of countless unschooled slaves, suddenly thrown on their own resources in their attempts to obtain food, shelter and clothing for their families. This appalling and pathetic situation prompted in Dr. Washington the desire to help these rural people and led to the inception in his mind of the Movable School idea. The plan has long since proved its worth and has passed far beyond the experimental stage."[68] Campbell's observation was indeed accurate (figure 14). When the Civil War ended in 1865, many black Southerners were encumbered with families having little or no access to sufficient necessities to keep them healthy (i.e., diseases, sanitation, and diet). These people were living in rural areas, engaged in farming or farming-related occupations, with little or no opportunity for economic growth or social advancement. Washington knew that for the poor of Macon County to become self-sufficient, there would have to be some mechanism that would teach them how to effectively manage their farms, livestock, and families. The mechanism of choice, the moveable school, would become the foundation for the nation's extension service. The development of this innovative contrivance by Washington took many years to complete.[69]

Within a few short years after the Civil War, the National Grange and the Farmers Alliance,[70] early agricultural societies, were developed to serve "as agricultural, educational, and social organizations for the benefit and comfort of the isolated rural classes."[71] The problem with these organizations in Alabama is that they were for white people only, resulting in the omission of almost half of the other farmers "by excluding blacks from membership."[72] This was a continuation of unfair practices that dominated national attitudes and politics, especially in the South, from before the end of the Civil War. Things were changing, but it would be a slow process.

On July 2, 1862, President Abraham Lincoln signed into law the Justin Smith Morrill and Land-Grant College Act, commonly known as the Morrill Act.[73] This act, while supposedly providing agricultural extension and re-

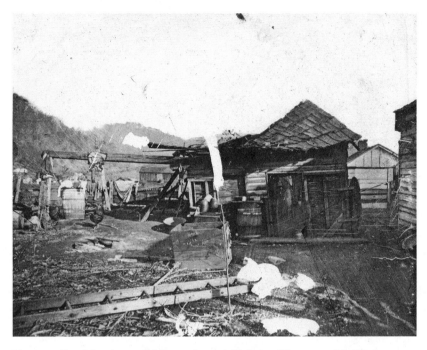

Figure 14. Rural farmhouse in Macon County, Alabama. (Courtesy of the Tuskegee University Archives)

search to farmers throughout the country, made no provisions for the use of land-grant funds[74] for black individuals. Although the majority of black people were still in slavery at the time and the act did not divide funds on racial lines, it would nonetheless serve as the foundation for allowing funds to be dispersed to black institutions in the future. Furthermore, the Morrill Act did have a provision for separate but equal facilities, but only a few Southern states took advantage of it.

Northern schools saw within the Morrill Act a prospect to allow both black people and women an opportunity to attend their land-grant schools, specifically for learning agriculture and the mechanical arts. Most Southern states did not want black students attending their schools so they sought other ways to meet the act's goals. The states would either give black students scholarships to attend a private black school, give money directly to the school, or build a school specifically for black people. The first land-grant institution for black students was Alcorn Agricultural and Mechanical College, now Alcorn University, founded in 1871 in Lorman, Mississippi. This was followed shortly by two other black institutions that received funds prior to 1890. They were Hampton University in Virginia, which would later give up its land-grant status to Virginia State, and Claflin University in South Carolina, which would later become South Carolina State. In fact, because of the first Morrill Act, a total of 16 black land-grant colleges were eventually founded:

1866: Lincoln University in Missouri
1871: Alcorn State University in Mississippi
1875: Alabama A&M University
1875: University of Arkansas at Pine Bluff
1878: Prairie View A&M University in Texas
1880: Southern University and A&M in Louisiana
1881: West Virginia State College
1882: Virginia State University
1886: Kentucky State University
1886: University of Maryland, Eastern Shore
1887: Florida A&M University
1891: Delaware State University
1891: North Carolina A&T University
1895: Fort Valley State University in Georgia
1896: South Carolina State University
1897: Langston University in Oklahoma

The first Morrill Act would lead to the Hatch Act of 1887 and the Second Morrill Act of 1890.

The Hatch Act[75] was indeed beneficial, especially to Tuskegee, because it established the National Agricultural Research System. This act gave federal funds, initially $15,000 each, to state land-grant colleges in order to create a series of agricultural experiment stations. These stations, in turn, were used to aid farmers by providing new information being developed regarding plant growth and livestock improvements. During this time, Tuskegee University, under Booker T. Washington, had begun a local extension work.

Within two days of his arrival at Tuskegee in 1881, Washington discovered his "school" consisted of a leaky frame structure offered by the Methodist Episcopal Church. The building seemed to be about to collapse at any moment and was accompanied by a nearby shanty whose condition was worse. There were no books, no slates, no desks, and no students. Washington borrowed a mule and wagon, and set out along the dusty roads to learn as much as possible about the people and their needs, and to let them know that a teacher, someone who cared, was among them. From that day on, Washington, because of his real concern for improving the conditions of the rural people, sought to extend the influence of his school into the rural communities of Macon County.[76]

Not only was he concerned with improving the quality of life for poor black farmers, but also he was concerned with the continued cycle of debt and poverty that was endemic to the sharecropper economy of the South. He reasoned that the norm for the federal government was to ignore their plight, while directing their attention to major metropolitan areas and the wants of special interest groups. The solution was to be accomplished through his vision for extension work. Simply put, farmers were to be instructed in a variety of topics and programs in order to help them become healthy and capable landowners.

At times, Washington rode his horse, Dexter; at other times he drove a wagon. What he found throughout the Black Belt Counties were "ramshackled cabins, occupied by poverty-stricken blacks who year after year struggled in cotton fields trying to eke out a miserable existence. After a long day's work, they came home to rest in the crude one or two room log cabins of rough pine slabs. In these shacks they slept and lived . . . In many of these shacks, there were as few as one or two beds with many of the families having a dozen persons ranging from infants to the old and decrepit. Pig pens were often at the door and a well from which they obtained water was down the hill below these pens. Windows, screens and steps were practically unknown. Many shacks had no toilet facilities whatever."[77]

As early as 1882, Washington was aware of the need for further assistance for the farmers and families of Macon County, far earlier than the date posited by James W. Smith. In an article titled "The Contributions of Black Americans to Agricultural Extension and Research," Smith noted: "As early as 1889 farmers' institutes and conferences were held in different states to provide black farmers with information related to the improvement of farm and home life. College experiment station personnel, physicians, and other specialists provided demonstrations and lectures to black farmers and homemakers in order to improve their health and happiness."[78] No doubt the poverty and unsanitary conditions of the rural farm families prompted Washington to act accordingly. His compassion and concern for his fellow man weighed heavily on his young psyche, prompting him to seek solutions available to him. The solutions developed due to the implementation of the Hatch Act at Tuskegee, providing a vehicle through which his ideas could be spread. This work would further develop with the advent of the second Morrill Act of 1890.

The second Morrill Act,[79] in conjunction with the Smith-Lever Act of May 8, 1914, further solidified black citizens into the system of cooperative extension and research. Under the second Morrill Act, federal funding was specifically earmarked for the creation of colleges for black students with the same legal status as the 1862 land-grant schools. Immediately, seventeen Southern and Border States took advantage of the funding and established the institutions commonly referred to today as 1890 land-grant colleges.

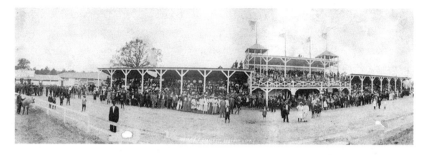

Figure 15. Tuskegee farmers' conference, 1912. (Courtesy of the Tuskegee University Archives)

The Smith–Lever Act of 1914[80] established a system of cooperative extension services connected to the land-grant universities. These services were multifaceted, providing a host of opportunities for rural people to learn about current developments in agriculture, home economics, public policy/government, leadership, 4-H, economic development, coastal issues (National Sea Grant College Program), and other related subjects.[81] However, under Washington, Tuskegee was already providing many of these services.

As early as 1888, Washington sought help, bringing in Charles W. Greene (1849–1926)[82] as superintendent of the school's farm. Immediately, Farmer Greene, as he was known by the locals, was a close confidant of Washington. Like his employer, Greene would travel by horse and buggy "to the county churches and homes and talk with the farmers and their wives about improved conditions which were in their power to make,"[83] probably often traveling and working in unison with Washington.

In 1890, Washington, with the aid of Greene and others, began holding monthly, small farmers meetings. These meetings, held on the campus, were meant to provide a platform for farmers to discuss their problems. Unfortunately, many of the farmers did not attend, fearing they were not on par with the "educated Negroes."[84] Furthermore, many found it difficult to arrange suitable transportation. In response, Washington either went out to see them or sent his teachers, in order to not only promote the school, but also to teach.

During the on-campus meetings, simple displays and exhibits of produce from the school's farm were made to show the farmers they could be more productive on smaller acreage at less expense. Other exhibits were intended to show farmers and their families how to make their homes more attractive and sanitary. The success of these early meetings resulted in larger, more intense opportunities, such as the Annual Negro Conference.[85]

By 1892, Tuskegee held its first Annual Negro Conference. The conference

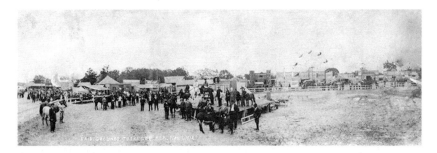

Figure 15. *Continued*

sought to accommodate people from all social strata and levels of education. Attendance at the first meeting was phenomenal. Over 400 men and women (including black and white attendees)[86] came to hear Washington conduct his programs "and discussions in such an informal and simple manner that the farmers were assured of their welcome to the school and readily made to feel that they were an integral part of the meetings." Eventually, the conference grew to over 2,000 attendees and evolved into a two-day event (figure 15).[87]

How important was this conference? T. M. Campbell notes that "In order to be on time, farmers left home as early as midnight prior to the meeting, in various types of vehicles and conveyances, including wagons drawn by oxen."[88] Washington was not timid when telling farm families about their need to change. Rather, what made him endearing to them was his ability to speak frankly without offending or embarrassing them. Because of his efforts, they did change, not only their farming habits, but also many changed their methods of food preparation and sanitary practices that had a direct correlation to their health. Campbell further notes: "This conference was the forerunner of the many modern farm congresses held at numerous agricultural colleges for both black and white people in various parts of the country."[89]

By 1896, a formal Department of Agriculture had been put in place, prompting Washington to recruit George Washington Carver as head of the school's Division of Agriculture. On February 15, 1897, Alabama approved an act establishing a branch agricultural experiment station and agricultural school for the "colored race" at Tuskegee.[90] Its purpose was to educate and train black students "so that the colored race may have an opportunity to acquire intelligent practical knowledge of agriculture in all various branches."[91] Carver was named director of the new experiment station, and six members of the faculty were assigned as staff.

Although the successes of the conferences were quickly evident, Washington felt there needed to be a method for teaching the locals throughout the

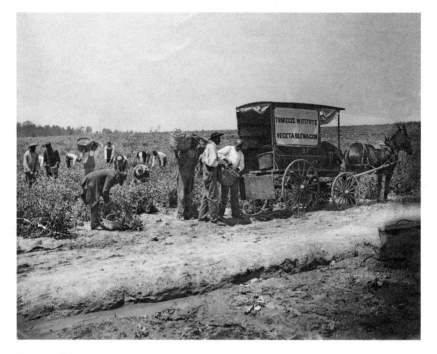

Figure 16. Tuskegee Institute vegetable wagon. (Courtesy of the Tuskegee University Archives)

year. In response, he sent out a simple, one-horse wagon called the "Tuskegee Institute vegetable wagon" (figure 16).[92]

Although this wagon was specifically for the teaching of important and useful agricultural practices, it would evolve into the Jesup Wagon. First, however, there was Carver and his buggy. From the time he came to Tuskegee, Carver continued the weekly trips begun by Washington, usually on the weekend, because he had other responsibilities to the school during the week. Carver traveled to rural communities where he made talks and gave instructive agricultural "demonstrations both varied and seasonal."[93]

Realizing most rural farm families would be found at church on Sunday, Carver utilized that time to teach them. Waiting until after the conclusion of church services, Carver proved to be "tremendously effective in capturing the interest and attention of these illiterate farmers. Such spare-time efforts, however, could hardly reach more than a small fraction of those who needed agricultural instruction."[94] This frustration led to the development of a more efficient method of meeting the masses, with more information and more demonstrations.

The Jesup Wagon

A Farmer's College on Wheels which educated the farmer in the field, while the Institute is teaching his children—a kindergarten method of making thrifty landowners out of hand-to-mouth negro tenants.
—Booker T. Washington (in Mayberry, *A Century of Agriculture in the 1890 Land-Grant Institutions and Tuskegee University-1890–1990*)

Interestingly, movable schools and demonstration work evolved as early as the early 1800s to solve these problems. Demonstration work had developed as a means for European progressive landowners, who were also often aristocrats, to improve their estate's production capabilities, the value of their estates, and their rental incomes. Movable schools, in which "itinerant agriculturists" traveled from farm to farm, became commonplace in France as early as 1837.[95] The concept of taking experts into the field to provide demonstrations to the farmers took hold as a result of the work of Iowa State University and Perry Holden in 1904. Called "Seed Corn Gospel Trains," Holden used train cars as traveling exhibits and lecture halls to demonstrate his methods to improve crop yields. No doubt, George Washington Carver's background with Iowa State aided him in the development of his demonstration wagon. However, the Jesup Wagon would prove to be much more than Holden's trains or France's "itinerant agriculturalists," and would provide much more information than Carver's simple buggy.

In 1904, Washington suggested to Carver that a wagon be outfitted as a "traveling agricultural school" to make regular trips into the countryside under a full-time operator. Carver declared the idea a "most excellent one" and immediately submitted a proposal for such a project.[96] Included in the proposal was a rough sketch (figure 17) of a "light, strong wagon body for either a one or two-horse wagon" that would open up to display all kinds of dairy equipment and large charts on "soil-building, orcharding, stock raising and all operations pertaining to the farm."[97] Carver suggested lectures be given on various phases of self-sufficient farming and soil examinations in an attempt to help farmers maximize crop output for various soils. Washington, looking at the broader picture, sought to teach about home life, specifically sanitation, better nutrition, general contentment, and community pride.

While Carver and his staff finalized the plans and prepared an estimate of the cost of an agricultural wagon, Washington went north to find the money to construct it. Morris K. Jesup, a New York banker and philanthropist, agreed to provide the $567.00[98] for the wagon and equipment, and to get the John F.

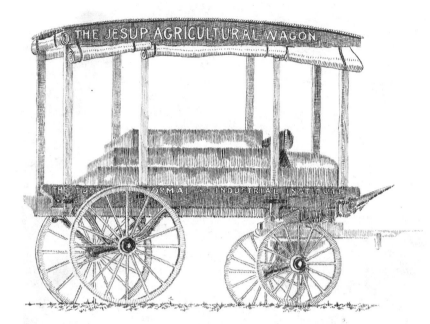

Figure 17. Carver's sketch of the Jesup Agricultural Wagon. (Courtesy of the Tuskegee University Archives)

Slater Fund to provide money for the wagon's operation. The wagon was constructed by students at Tuskegee (figure 18) and began its inaugural trips May 24, 1906.

The Jesup Agricultural Wagon, called by Washington the "Farmers' College on Wheels," began its trips into the rural areas of the county, with George Bridgeforth[99] as the first operator. Specifically, the wagon (figure 19) carried different kinds of plows and planters, a cultivator, a cotton chopper, a variety of seeds, samples of fertilizers, a revolving churn, a butter mold, a cream separator, a milk tester, and other appliances useful in making practical demonstrations. It further had the advantage of carrying scientific agriculture directly to the farmers working in the field. After making the rounds of the small and large farms of a community, the "movable school" was located at a central point and conducted an open-air demonstration for a gathering of farmers and their families. During the summer of 1906, the school on wheels reached over 2,000 people a month and attracted attention all over the state. White farmers began attending the meetings, and some of them who owned large plantations invited the Jesup Wagon to visit their black tenants.[100] It became obvious to Washington this innovation was one of his greatest, and it would "do much to break through

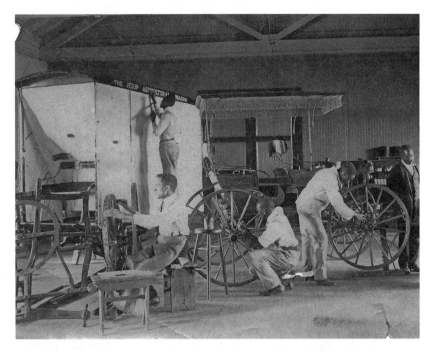

Figure 18. Students constructing the Jesup Wagon. (Courtesy of the Tuskegee University Archives)

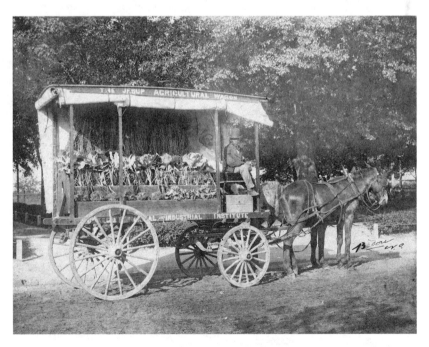

Figure 19. The Jesup Wagon in use. (Courtesy of the Tuskegee University Archives)

the hard crust of custom and prepare for a new agricultural era."[101] The equipment and demonstrations varied according to the season.[102]

The importance of the Jesup Wagon cannot be overstated, but it was not readily accepted within every community. Campbell described one instance where he:

> came to a community where the usual summer revival, sometimes referred to as a "protracted meeting," was in session at the local church. Upon learning that many of the people had gathered there, I sought to take advantage of the gathering by driving my wagon to the church grove. I unhitched the team, arranged my equipment in exhibit fashion and sent an associate into the church to ask the preacher to announce that when the service was concluded, I would be on the outside and would like to give a demonstration and make some remarks. The people came out in large numbers and, out of curiosity, looked at the large wagon and its driver, but did not remain for my demonstration. My associate informed me, to my surprise, that before he could get a chance to speak, the preacher asked his congregation to rise, and just before the benediction was pronounced said: "I see the Tuskegee farm wagon has just drove up on the outside, and I don't know what they plan to do, but I just lak [sic] to say to the members of this church that we can't afford to engage in worldly affairs while we are busy engaged in saving souls, and I advise you not to take up any time with the wagon." He also cautioned the people to "watch those silver tongued speakers and the man with a pencil behind his ear."[103]

Attitudes soon changed, and the Jesup Wagon became the talk of the region. Campbell further relates anecdotally the drastic change in these attitudes. In a letter from L. W. Owens, an educated rural minister, Campbell noted how Owens

> wondered what could really happen at 8:00 o'clock in the morning with grown-ups. On reaching the house, I found myself completely upset in my imagination and wholly out of harmony with the work. Everybody was in work clothes and too busy to see me. The class in terracing was in a near-by field where the farmers were being given lessons in the use of the tripod and target in running terraces. Another class was standing around a large barrel where they were learning how to make and apply whitewash and how to mix stains. Other classes were being taught in rug-making, the candling of eggs, dyeing, care of the sick room, building poultry houses and sanitary toilets, soap making, lawn building. Every-

thing possible was being taught that makes rural life a life of happiness and contentment. Of course this was my first day's experience in a Movable School. The second day I was there on time with my old discarded hand saw and suit of overalls which fitted me for the occasion.[104]

The juxtaposition between the two farmers' accounts is significant, no doubt reflecting how quickly the Jesup Wagon was accepted.

During a visit to Tuskegee in the fall of 1906, Dr. Seaman A. Knapp, special agent in charge of Farmers Cooperative Demonstration work for the United States Department of Agriculture (USDA), discussed the possibilities of developing a cooperative demonstration program for black farmers in the South. In a deft move, Washington seized this opportunity to link Tuskegee's extension work with that of the federal government. Dr. Knapp, using funds provided by the General Education Board,[105] and Booker T. Washington, with money from the Slater Fund,[106] agreed to share the expenses for employing someone to operate the Jesup Wagon. This individual was to conduct demonstration work in Macon and surrounding counties. In response to that need, T. M. Campbell, a recent graduate in agriculture from Tuskegee, was hired on November 12, 1906.[107]

The Jesup Wagon continued to be successful and experience growth. After the passage of the Smith-Lever Act in 1914, Alabama Polytechnic Institute (API) at Auburn (now called Auburn University) assumed responsibility for all extension work in agriculture and home economics in Alabama. In addition to the male agent, a female home demonstration agent was added in order to help the wives and women on the rural farm.[108] These new agents were responsible for teaching young girls and women "how to make and use home conveniences, how to care for poultry, cook, sew, can, and conduct the home on a more healthful and economic basis."[109]

The Jesup Wagon did have its limitations. Due to poor roads, inaccessible farms, and increasing distances brought on by demand for programs and demonstrations in other counties, other solutions were sought to alleviate the increased time and cost the project was to Tuskegee. Campbell notes, "a system was adopted whereby the agents traveled by train from headquarters to the nearest railroad station. The equipment was placed in trunks and checked as baggage. Farmers would drive us from the stations to the different communities."[110] Unfortunately, even this solution proved problematic. It cost money to hire transport from the train stations to the location where the demonstrations would take place. Sometimes agents could teach from the trains, but participation was limited because those who needed help lived away and did not have adequate transportation. It became more apparent that a truck needed to be purchased in order to overcome these hindrances.

Even during Washington's waning years he never gave up his visits to the homes of the rural farmers. His last rural trip occurred in 1914, in which he insisted "that the houses along the roads traveled by the 'Washington Party' be whitewashed, the yards cleaned, and fences repaired in advance of their coming" (figure 20). He also urged the farmers to grow their own foodstuffs and have some produce on exhibit along the roadside in front of their houses . . . In his speeches; he always admonished his hearers to 'quit living out of tin cans and paper bags.'"[111] His intentions were always toward the betterment, both physically and mentally, of these people.

The Knapp Agricultural Truck

> If a few of the millions that are spent, and I think sometimes partially
> wasted, on the wealthier classes, in so called higher education, could be
> spent remodeling the homes of the poor and changing their view points
> [*sic*] it would be a great and lasting benefit to the world!
> —Seaman A. Knapp, Special Agent, Farmer's Cooperative
> Demonstration Work, USDA (Letter from Dr. Seaman
> Knapp to George Washington Carver, February 20, 1907).

After API took over extension work within the state, the needs for farmers in Macon and surrounding counties did not abate. Funding for extension work was limited, especially amongst black farmers. Booker T. Washington addressed the disparities of the Smith-Lever Act, noting that of the $100,280.00 in funds allocated to the state in 1914, "the colored people receive only $22,500.00." [112] He further reasoned that this small amount made "it impossible to do any effective and practical work for the colored farmers except it is done through and by colored people themselves."[113]

By 1918, the necessity for more reliable transportation to be used in the Tuskegee extension work became more apparent. The Jesup Wagon had become obsolete and fallen into disrepair (figure 21). An appeal was made to Dr. J. F. Duggar, then state director of extension in Alabama, in order to procure funds for a truck to be used for agriculture demonstration projects. The Ford[114] truck (figure 22) was named the "Knapp Agricultural Truck" (also called the Knapp Wagon) in honor of Dr. Seaman A. Knapp, founder of farm demonstration work in America.

This new vehicle proved to be a boon to the work, making it possible to cover more territory and carry additional workers and equipment. Although this new vehicle utilized some of the same types of demonstration projects, its size allowed for increased displays. Interestingly, enlarged coverage by the Jesup Wagon and later the Knapp Wagon "revealed that a tremendous amount

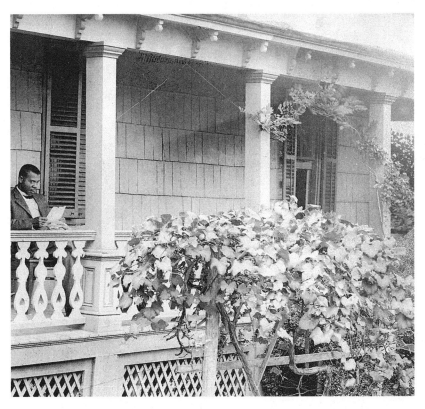

Figure 20. Booker T. Washington reading on a farmer's quiet porch. (Courtesy of the Tuskegee University Archives)

of sickness prevailed in a large number of the homes in every community visited."[115] Booker T. Washington recognized the health disparities amongst poor black farm families, and had already put into place health-care efforts on the campus and within the local community. These rural farmers suffered from a wide range of health maladies, "including malaria, typhoid fever, hookworm disease, pellagra, and venereal disease, along with malnutrition and high infant and maternal mortality rates."[116] But the efforts of the various extension projects drew further attention to how widespread this need was; it was greater than just Macon County and Tuskegee University. This proved a great concern for the leadership at Tuskegee.

In an attempt to address this need, in 1920, a registered nurse was appointed to look into the personal health of the people and the sanitation of their homes and surroundings, and incidentally to help guard against disease. The nurse's salary was to be paid jointly by Tuskegee and the Alabama State Health De-

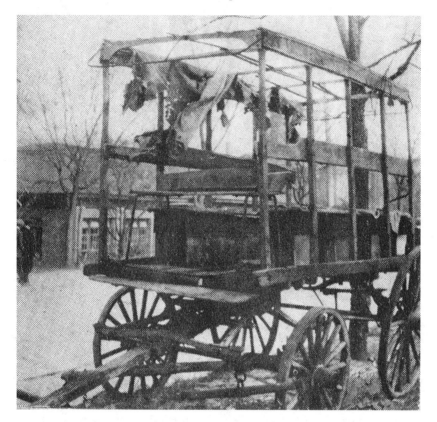

Figure 21. The Jesup Wagon in disrepair. (Courtesy of the Tuskegee University Archives)

partment. Uva M. Hester, a Tuskegee graduate, was hired for the position and immediately thrust into situations no doubt akin to working in a battlefield triage. Her first report, written after just one week of work in Montgomery County, Alabama, illustrates how difficult health care was amongst the poor black farm families: "Tuesday: I visited a young woman who had been bed-ridden with tuberculosis for more than a year. There are two openings on her chest and one in the side from which pus constantly streams. In addition, there is a bedsore on the lower part of the back as large as one's hand. There were no sheets on the bed. In the absence of a basin or bowl for bathing the patient, a kitchen utensil was used. The sores had only a patch of cloth plastered over them. No effort was made to protect the patient from the flies that swarmed around her. The patient lives near a dairy but is not furnished with milk."[117]

But the Movable School and its nurse faced additional challenges. Although not entirely unexpected, superstitions and home remedies[118] proved difficult to overcome before Hester's advice was accepted and followed. Extension Agent T. M. Campbell reported: "The Movable School force once went into a com-

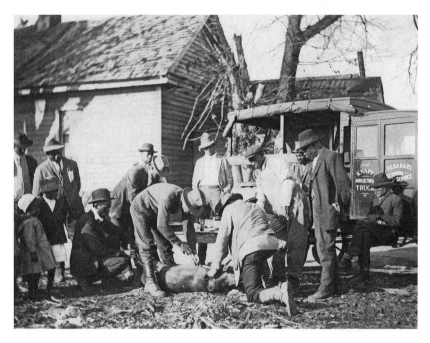

Figure 22. A farm hog being inoculated by workers from the Knapp Agricultural Truck. (Courtesy of the Tuskegee University Archives)

munity just after a voodoo man[119] had 'worked' it to his financial gain. He had been able to dispose of a large number of 'wonder beans,' merely buckeyes, at a dollar each. Many Negroes bought these beans on the assurance that if they were worn about the necks, no bodily harm could come to them. In making one of her usual rounds, our nurse found in one home the mother smoking her two children with tar, feathers, and old shoes. On being asked why she did this, she said her children had been 'running at the noses' all winter and she remembered that when she was a child, her father always smoked the mules and it helped them so she thought she would try it on her children."[120]

Hester's observations led to specific responses to the needs of the rural farm families, especially children. Campbell reports that she advised them on sanitary practices in order to combat the spreading of diseases, as well as the importance of proper nutrition in maintaining good health. If immediate treatments proved inadequate, she would refer them to a local physician or the John A. Andrew Memorial Hospital in Tuskegee.

After five years of countless miles on poor roads, the Knapp Wagon became too decrepit to operate. It had traveled not only throughout Macon and adjacent counties, but beyond to Mississippi and Georgia. Its fame had spread far beyond the original intent of Booker T. Washington and those that followed. The needs remained such that in 1923, a new and larger truck was acquired.

"Booker Washington On Wheels"

A GREAT CAMPAIGN HAS BEEN LAUNCHED BY THE
FARMERS OF ALABAMA TO BUILD AN

Agricultual Motor Truck

TO THE MEMORY OF THE LATE BOOKER WASHING-
TON, FOR THE PURPOSE OF TRAVELING AMONG THE
COLORED FARMERS TO GIVE FIRST-HAND INFORMA-
TION IN DAIRYING, LIVESTOCK RAISING, GARDEN-
ING AND ALL LINES TOUCHING THE LIFE OF THE
COLORED FARMERS.

Each County in which "Extension Workers" are employed has been assessed for building and maintaining the
"Truck."

BULLOCK COUNTY'S QUOTA IS $175.00

Campaign begins January 14, 1922. I will call on every
Business Man, Farmer, Firm, Corporation, Church, School,
Teacher, Minister and Fraternal Organization for a donation
to such a worthy cause.

Every person donating will be given Free a beautiful
Portrait of the late Booker Washington. Every Patriotic
Citizen will help to put Agriculture in Bullock County on a
paying basis.

Harry Sims of Tuskegee Institute has been selected as
custodian of all Funds.

M. B. IVY,

Local Dem. Agt.

HERALD, UNION SPRINGS, ALA.

Figure 23. Flyer soliciting funds for a new truck. (Courtesy of the Tuskegee University Archives)

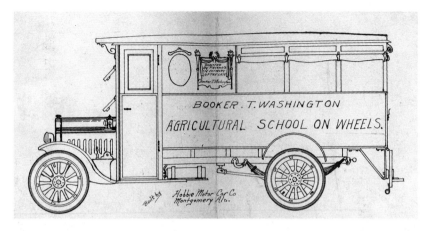

Figure 24. Sketch of Booker T. Washington Agricultural School on Wheels. (Courtesy of the Tuskegee University Archives)

The Booker T. Washington Agricultural School on Wheels

A man is not fit to work with the country people unless he has smelled the soil and can converse with them in their own lingo.

—Honorable Henry Wallace, Secretary of Agriculture
(in Virginia Lantz Denton, *Booker T. Washington and the Adult Education Movement*)

Due to the dilapidated state of the Knapp Wagon, a new mode of transportation was sought in order to reach more people with more information. In 1923, more than 30,000 supporters of this important work, many of them the African American farmers who had been helped by the Movable School, contributed $5,000 to purchase a new vehicle (figure 23). Built by the Hobby Motor Company of Montgomery, Alabama, the Booker T. Washington Agricultural School on Wheels (figure 24), as it was aptly named, was presented at the Thirty-Second Annual Tuskegee Negro Conference.

This third and final Movable School brought with it spraying equipment, a set of carpenter's tools, a milk tester, an inoculating set for vaccinating livestock, a lighting plant for generating electricity on the farm, a moving picture projector, cameras, a sewing machine, an electric iron, a baby's bathtub, a set of baby's clothes, a medicine cabinet, kitchen utensils, and playground apparatus for recreational games. The Moveable School was staffed with a farm demonstration agent, a home agent, and a registered nurse.

The most significant difference between this wagon (figure 25) and the previous schools' was the outcome intended for farmers and their families. Instead

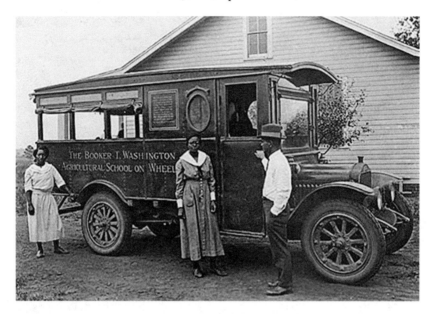

Figure 25. The Booker T. Washington Agricultural School on Wheels with a farm agent, home agent, and nurse. (Courtesy of the Tuskegee University Archives)

of demonstrations held in towns or communities, agents would locate at a specific farm convenient for others to visit. Individuals, both men and women, came to these functions to learn in the best possible format. The farm agent would conduct hands-on demonstrations in the field or barn. Techniques for making farm life more streamlined and modern were emphasized. The home agent worked to show women how to can, clean, and accomplish domestic chores that made the home more healthful and economically sufficient. The nurse concentrated on hygiene, sanitation, and the care of the sick. All of these worked in tandem to make their lives better.

Some of the farms they visited were large and very fertile. Some farmers had large holdings of livestock and even had tenants to work the land, yet they lived in houses that were little better than those of the tenants. T. M. Campbell related the following: "In one community we found a farmer who owned 300 acres of land and had just bargained for 200 acres more. He had a splendid stock barn, but his home consisted of two small rooms, no window lights, no steps to either of the two outer doors, and no fence of any kind about the yard. Although there were eleven children in the family, there was no toilet on the place."[121] Although Booker T. Washington and others saw these farms as positive examples (excluding the houses), they desired to use the poorest farms, with dilapidated barns, house, yards, and fields for their demonstrations. The poorer farms were representative of the average type of farm found throughout the South.

Having a registered nurse proved to be advantageous for a variety of issues, such as "home sanitation . . . child welfare, screening the home, caring for the patient in the home, eradication of vermin and directing of severe cases of illness to the community physician."[122] Campbell emphasized: "Failure to appreciate the proverbial 'an ounce of prevention is better than a pound of cure.' The ignorant rural Negro often allows his home to become or remain a run down shack, around which health conditions become so terrible that the way is paved for the most ravaging diseases. As a result he is obliged to pay excessive doctor bills, and experiences a high mortality among the members of his family. It is through these and many other similar deplorable conditions that the Movable School force attempts to work its way to the bottom of the rural Negro's problem."[123] He concluded, "The South must also give more attention to the health of rural Negroes. Possibly the most neglected phase of public service today among them is sanitation and simple health instruction. Negro farmers are not likely to give much attention to hogs stricken with cholera, nor to weevil-infested cotton, when their families are suffering from tuberculosis, typhoid, malaria and hookworm disease. The squalor, filth, disease and dilapidation of their surroundings reflect not only upon them, but upon the whole South; and this condition constitutes not only a Negro problem, nor a Southern problem, but a national one."[124]

The Movable School was retired from service in 1944 due to the development of a permanent workforce of Cooperative Extension Agents throughout the South. The school, in all of its incarnations, continued the vision of Booker T. Washington to make things better for the people of the South. Even though its primary thrust was to aid black farm families, white people participated and were equal recipients of the work. Men and women became healthier and more self-sufficient, while their quality of life increased.

2
Health Education and Outreach Expands

As things are happening in the world today, America has in the Negro an asset of indispensible value. Bound together by ties of common suffering and sacrifice in times of distress it is unthinkable that these two elements should be anything else than allies in whatever undertaking they may face in the future. Meanwhile, nothing can contribute more toward the establishment of our national welfare than the continued effort to realize for the humblest in our national life, whether black or white, that full measure of justice and equal opportunity for which America stands as a symbol before the world. To this task thousands of the noblest spirits in our country are dedicated. It is such as thee that make all, regardless of race, proud to be an American.

—Robert Moton (1929)

Under Tuskegee University's second and third presidents, Robert Moton and Frederick D. Patterson, health care at Tuskegee continued Washington's vision with increased opportunities at the John A. Andrew Memorial Hospital and outreach programs such as the National Negro Health Week. Moton staunchly supported the work, bringing health care for black communities to the national forefront, while Patterson sought to provide a place for black patients to come for instruction and treatment. Some critically important programs were established during this period that provided support for the community health needs.

Tuskegee Institute Chapter of the American Red Cross

Early during the tenure of Moton, the university had "the unique privilege of being the only regularly chartered Red Cross chapter for Negroes, not only in the United States, but the only one of purely Negro membership in the world."[1] Founded in 1918, this chapter was established at a time when many doubted the ability of black Americans to participate in the nation's defense, let alone in disaster relief. This chapter was founded within two decades of the beginning of the administering body.

Founded by Clara Barton and friends in Washington, DC, on May 21, 1881, the American Red Cross received its first charter from Congress in 1900 and a

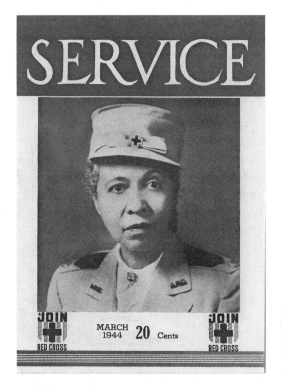

Figure 26. Bess Bolden Walcott featured on a 1944 Red Cross poster. (Courtesy of the Tuskegee University Archives)

second in 1905. The purpose of the organization "included giving relief to and serving as a medium of communication between members of the American armed forces and their families and providing national and international disaster relief and mitigation."[2] These principles coincided with those of Tuskegee University, which sought to "continue to grow in its field of usefulness to the Negro race."

The chapter was overseen by executive secretary Bess Bolden Walcott (1886–1988) (figure 26) who served in that position for more than thirty years. Born in Xenia, Ohio, Walcott was recruited by Booker T. Washington from Oberlin College as a librarian, later serving in a variety of positions including as teacher and administrator. Although her long life was replete with numerous awards and commendations for a variety of accomplishments, it was her work with the American Red Cross at which she most excelled.

In 1924, Tuskegee's chapter opened one of the first health centers in the South to be staffed by a public health nurse. Later, during the Great Depression, her efforts procured a grant from the American Red Cross to distribute food and other necessities to destitute Southern black farm families. And during the Second World War Walcott became the first black woman to become a

Red Cross acting field director. Serving from 1941 to 1942, she worked in support of the famed Tuskegee Airmen by promoting the war effort through war bonds and press releases that chronicled their progress. After the war, she was reappointed acting field director (1946–1947) in order to oversee the needs of returning veterans.

The VA Hospital at Tuskegee

Following World War I, the Treasury Department Hospitalization Committee found it was almost impossible to secure proper treatment for black soldiers, especially in the South, thus "the federal government decided to open a hospital for black veterans because of the discrimination they faced at existing"[3] hospitals. Heeding outcries from a variety of organizations such as the NAACP, the Veterans Administration (VA) sought locations to build hospitals specifically for black veterans. Tuskegee University agreed to donate 300 acres for just such a hospital.[4] The VA Hospital[5] located at the edge of Tuskegee University's campus was a segregated but well-equipped institution with an all-black staff that included twenty-two physicians.[6]

Initially, in order to garner their support, white residents of Macon County were told by US officials the hospital would be staffed and controlled by white personnel. Robert Moton, on the other hand, desired black administrators to be in control in order to provide jobs for black doctors and nurses. This would also afford a venue for those in control "to demonstrate black managerial ability."[7] Moton, assisted by the influential black press, the Urban League, and the NAACP, pressured VA officials, including President Warren G. Harding, seeking to develop an all-black staff in the hospital.[8] White people countered by mobilizing to push for white control.

The hospital, constructed at a cost of 2.5 million dollars, consisted of twenty-seven buildings covering 464 acres. The dedication ceremony of the hospital, which was then known as the Hospital for Sick and Injured World War Veterans, occurred on February 23, 1923. The institution was passed in authority from the US Treasury to the US Veterans Bureau (which in July 1930 became the Veterans Authority).[9] Regarding this time, author Linda McMurray wrote: "Tuskegee whites quickly mobilized to ensure that the original promise of white control was realized. When the hospital opened they seemed to have won, for it was staffed mainly by whites. Black protest accelerated, resulting in increased racial tension in Tuskegee. Moton left town and went to work behind the scenes, as Washington often had in civil rights matters."[10] President Harding capitulated, ordering the immediate hiring of black employees in all positions at the hospital, thereby prompting the Ku Klux Klan to plan a march in retaliation. Black citizens from all across the state came in defense of the changes. In the end, the VA Hospital in Tuskegee became an all-black institution. The transition was completed on July 7, 1924, and was a significant victory for black people everywhere, further illustrating the growth and newfound power of black resistance to segregationist policies.[11]

Shirley Bealer, acting director of the Central Alabama Veterans Health Care System, on occasion of the Tuskegee VA Hospital's 85th anniversary, noted: "In 1923, young African American health care professionals were drawn to Tuskegee. They knew the nation would take stock in their ability and they knew they would not only be able to provide care for black veterans, but they would also serve as beacons for other young African Americans. Their commitment and professionalism would be scrutinized, measured and compared to the highest standards."[12] Those who came to the VA to work were committed to its success, some serving their entire careers. Dr. Toussaint T. Tildon,[13] a psychiatrist and one of the first six African American doctors, would go on to serve at the hospital for thirty-four years, serving nine years as director.

Veterans, who came from all over the country to the VA for treatment and rehabilitation, were often there for long periods of time. To meet their needs, the VA Hospital complex was built as a small, self-contained city. It had a complete hospital with surgery, physical therapy, occupational therapy, and counseling. Furthermore, in addition to apartments, there was a bowling alley, barber shop, gift shop, snack shop, laundry, library, movie theater, baseball field, golf course, and tennis courts. The hospital also possessed a fire department with a water tower providing its own water supply.

Establishment of the Macon County Health Department, 1928

At the turn of the twentieth century, "there were few independent Negro farmers in the South. The economic position of the southern rural Negro was pitiably bad."[14] To reach a rural farmer, one had to travel by horseback or horse and buggy or go by foot. News that traveled by mail required many citizens to make their "mark upon documents which they could not read."[15]

Fortunately, the economic blow delivered by the Great Depression was not as severe in Macon County as it was in some other Alabama counties. This was due to the presence of the Tuskegee VA Hospital and Tuskegee University, both of which offered employment to many in the immediate area. The economy was further stimulated by university students and staff personnel who bought from both black and white businesses.[16] Despite economic interaction, racial discrimination still prevailed. Health care, like the schools, was segregated and not equal.

Macon County Hospital,[17] a small thirty-bed, poorly equipped building, located adjacent to Tuskegee Lake, admitted only white patients. Conversely, John A. Andrew Memorial Hospital (JAAMH), having approximately one hundred and twenty beds, was a modern facility located on the campus of Tuskegee University. It provided quality health care for black patients, including all amenities that insured a wholesome and pleasant environment for the sick.[18] For approximately twenty-seven years, JAAMH was the only facility dedicated to the hospitalization of black patients within East Central Alabama.

During this time there were no formalized State Health Department facilities within Macon County. The Alabama State Department of Public Health was organized in 1896 due to increased numbers of cases of yellow fever, pneumonia, and tuberculosis within the state.[19] It was not until 1917 that legislation paved the way for the institution of public health services or health departments at the county level. Eleven years later, on April 1, 1928, the Macon County Health Department was established.

The purpose of public health services was for the improvement and protection of the public's health through disease prevention, regardless of social circumstances or the ability to pay. They were not hospitals, although they could refer patients to doctors or hospitals as needed. Beyond providing health assessment information to the community, they also provided information for disease prevention and enforced health regulations.[20] Meanwhile, JAAMH continued to provide general and surgical medical services to black patients in Macon and surrounding counties.[21] The support of both Robert Moton and other leaders at Tuskegee for the hospital to serve as a training ground for black doctors and nurses was not abated, but increased. There were, however, other issues that appear to some to have tainted the legacies in research and health care of Moton (and Patterson),[22] and therefore Tuskegee.

Eugenics and Tuskegee

At approximately the same time as the beginning of what would be known as the Tuskegee Syphilis Study, another issue, just as critical, serious, and pathological, was gaining a larger foothold on the methodology of researchers in the health/medical field. Eugenics,[23] the study of physiological variations in an attempt to prove hereditary differences between the races, had been growing in popularity throughout the early 1900s, and Tuskegee was involved as a proving ground.[24]

As early as 1913, Booker T. Washington approached Charles Davenport (1866–1944)[25] of the Carnegie Institution at Cold Spring Harbor, New York, a leading eugenicist, inviting him to come "study our teachers and students."[26]

Robert Norrell, author of *Up from History: The Life of Booker T. Washington*,[27] posits he probably "hoped measures of his students would demonstrate they were perfectly healthy and not about to 'wither away,' an idea that was pushed by some eugenicists who saw blacks as inferior."[28] Davenport, however, did not get to make that trip before Washington died in November 1915.

It was not until 1932 that Davenport would finally get the opportunity to visit Tuskegee and conduct his research. Then President Robert Moton permitted Davenport to come, but Davenport was at Tuskegee only a short while when he was followed by his colleague and confidant Morris Steggerda (1900–1950)[29] who would continue to collect data for the remainder of the study. Steggerda, like Davenport, worked at the Carnegie Institution and had been conducting eugenic research in the Yucatán of Mexico as well as Jamaica in the Caribbean.

Moton had asked Davenport for a plan of study, no doubt accepting him based on his impeccable qualifications from the National Academy of Sciences, the American Association for the Advancement of Science, and the US Army. This respectability, coupled with the fact there was, at that time, "nothing inherently suspect about anthropometry,[30] and it was accepted as part of scientific study in the U.S. for more than a generation. It had been used by racists and anti-racists alike."[31] The plan of study probably gave Moton some insight into the methods, and possibly the motives, which would be applied during the project. Moton and the administration would have utilized the plan of study in order to determine not only who would be assisting, but also who would be studied.

Davenport originally worked with Louise Atkins, of the Physical Education Department.[32] Following Steggerda's appointment to the study, Atkins continued her involvement because she knew "what the project implie[d]." Although two coaches, Cleve Abbott (1892–1955)[33] and Christine Petty,[34] were later assigned to work with the project, it appears that individuals from the Physical Education Department were the primary assistants with the early field work. Football coach Abbott, one of the most successful coaches of the time, and women's track and field coach Petty no doubt would have provided Steggerda with impressive athletic specimens to be measured and recorded. Record-breaking 100-meter sprinter (1938–1939) Mozelle Ellerbe of Tuskegee was measured as an example of the black race's finest.

Initially, Davenport planned for the study to last twelve years,[35] during which he anticipated collecting data on subjects from first grade through high school. In fact, the study was not to be limited to Tuskegee University, but would comprise schools throughout Macon County, including the local Children's House on Tuskegee's campus.[36] Studies were completed over 200 indi-

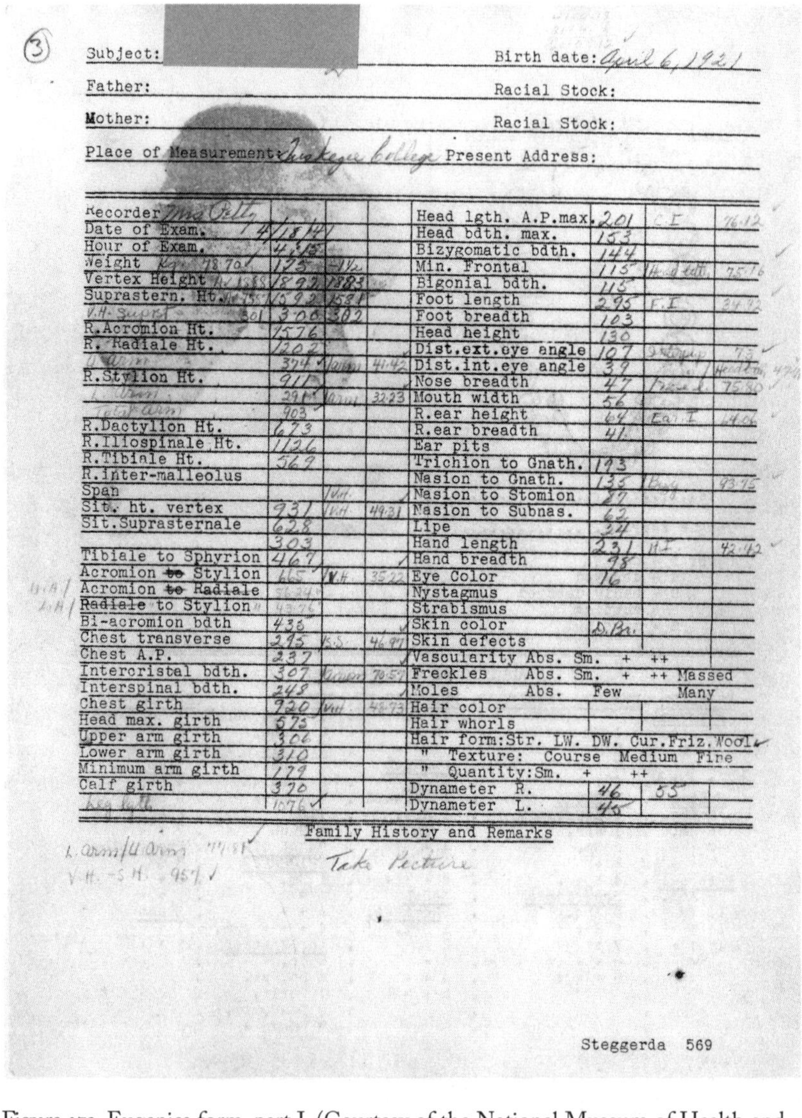

Figure 27a. Eugenics form, part I. (Courtesy of the National Museum of Health and Medicine)

viduals, which were documented on special forms that often included a photograph (figures 27a and 27b[37]).[38]

In a letter to Steggerda, Moton gave permission for him to "conduct the tests here at the Institute during March" of 1934.[39] Steggerda actually arrived on March 28, where he worked for the next few weeks. It is during this time Steggerda trained his assistants to take measurements of the children.[40] A manual

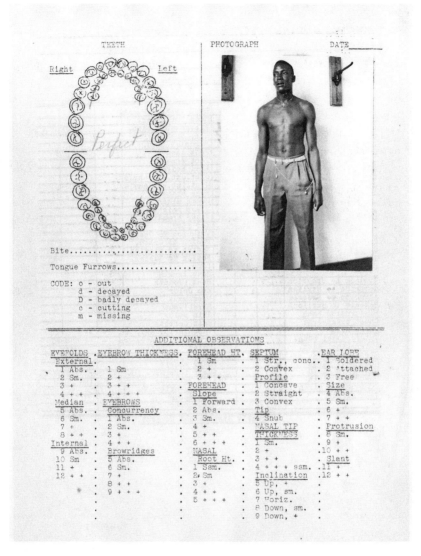

Figure 27b. Eugenics form, part II. (Courtesy of the National Museum of Health and Medicine)

was provided detailing how measurements were to be made "with pictures to illustrate the process, sketches of the instruments used and data collection blanks."[41] The detailed physiological studies included, but were not limited to, brow size, depth of nostrils, and length of ear lobes, a total of sixty-five different measurements. Petty, the women's coach, later acted as the study coordinator, and became the main link between Steggerda and the students. The study actually began before Petty's employment in 1936;[42] it appears Atkins was no longer employed at Tuskegee after 1935.

The majority of the study actually occurred during the presidency of Frederick D. Patterson. Patterson's tenure began in 1935 and continued throughout the rest of the study. Although there is very little documentation between the Tuskegee administration and Steggerda, no doubt there was some discussion behind the scenes. Patterson allowed the study to continue unabated.

So, why did the study continue at Tuskegee, even though eugenics was becoming increasingly less accepted during the late 1930s?[43] The Tuskegee administration was filled with capable and intelligent men that no doubt continued to support the study as an opportunity to show there was no significant physical difference between black and white people, and that they were just as capable as their white counterparts, despite what some "respectable" scientists might have speculated.

The faultiness of Davenport's and Steggerda's reports was significant. According to eugenic ideology, most of the testing was based on bad assumptions and failed to take into consideration physiological similarities among the races. Author Charles E. Rosenberg notes, "man is not an ideal experimental animal, and the tools and concepts of biology at the turn of the century were not equal to unraveling the complexities of human genetics" and "the inheritance of human traits made an objective study of these traits impossible."[44] Participants were selectively chosen based on preconceived notions of what "pure blacks" looked like, while rejecting some participants based on their similarities to what "pure whites" looked like. People of mixed-race descent and any who were perceived as having some "white" ancestry were rejected from the study.[45]

Steggerda relied on black participants to take the measurements that were meant to prove their own inferiority. This type of research further reveals the flaws of the study.[46] Making the proper measurements within the established guidelines provided by Davenport and later Steggerda required intense concentration, careful observation, intellectual honesty, and comprehension of what was mandatory for meeting the requirements of the established standards. The accomplishment of these requirements further negated the idea of black inferiority, as the black scientists that collected the data at Tuskegee were just as capable as their white counterparts.

Although Davenport planned for the study to span twelve years, the Carnegie Institution withdrew its support in 1940 from the eugenics program at Cold Spring Harbor, prompting the work at Tuskegee to end in 1942 after approximately ten years. Steggerda would go on to publish at least three articles utilizing data acquired at Tuskegee. By then, very little support was given to these studies, especially after the rise of Nazism and their promotion of eugenics research.

Continued Support and Training

Black participation within the medical community should not be perceived as limited to the number of doctors available within the United States prior to the 1950s. By 1947, only 49 of the 119 graduates of Howard University and Meharry Medical College were allowed internships at eight white hospitals. In 1948, there were 1,258 graduates from southern medical schools, and only 56 of them were black; all those were students at Meharry.[47] In response to this blatant shortage, and realizing the need for black physicians to have a place to go for internships and residencies (which were required in order to receive a license to practice medicine),[48] Frederick D. Patterson, president of Tuskegee University noted: "As president, I have been in conference with officials of the State of Alabama seeking to establish relationships which will insure that funds spent and programs developed in the future by the state for training nurses and physicians will be placed at this institution (i.e. Tuskegee University)."[49] Patterson voiced a growing concern he felt could only be resolved through the use of Tuskegee University's medical facilities, including the nearby Veterans Hospital (Number 91),[50] as a place for internships and residencies.

Furthermore, in an article published in the *New York Times*, Dr. Howard Rusk wrote, "In 1947, there were only 93 Negro students in twenty predominately white medical schools."[51] By 1956, the number had increased to 216 black students in forty-eight predominately white medical schools. Following criticism of admission policies at medical schools by black medical leaders and lay agencies, and the decisions by the Supreme Court in the Gaines and Sipuel cases, medical schools in Arkansas, Texas, and St. Louis opened their doors to black students. By 1971, segregation in medical schools had all but ended.[52]

Internships for medical school graduates were also limited. In 1940, only two white institutions provided them to black candidates on a quota basis, namely City Hospital in Cleveland, Ohio, and Harlem Hospital in New York City. At the same time, black hospitals that provided internships included Freedman's in Washington, DC; Provident Hospital of Cook County, in Chicago, Illinois; General Hospital No. 2, Kansas City, Kansas;[53] and Homer G. Phillips in St. Louis. Other black hospitals, which offered non-American Medical Association sanctioned internships, were John A. Andrew Memorial Hospital (figure 28) at Tuskegee University and Mercy-Douglas in Philadelphia, Pennsylvania.

Specialty training in the major subdivisions of medicine and surgery was practically nonexistent outside of the above-mentioned black hospitals. In 1940, for example, there was no institution that offered black students approved training in orthopedics. In 1941, Dr. Charles R. Drew was appointed chief of surgery at Howard University Medical School and through his efforts an approved Orthopedic Residency was established under the directorship of Dr.

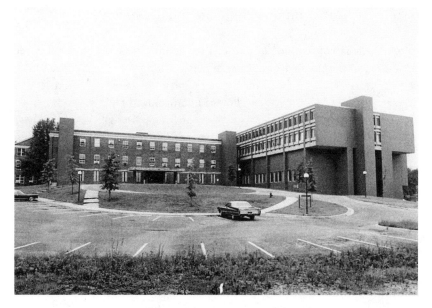

Figure 28. John A. Andrew Memorial Hospital. (Courtesy of the Tuskegee University Archives)

Julius Neviaser, chief of orthopedics at George Washington University, Washington, DC. The first black certified orthopedist in the country, Dr. James R. Gladden (certified in 1949), was a product of this program.

The second black orthopedist to be certified was Dr. John F. Hume (1915–2004),[54] also a product of the Howard University program. After completion of his residency and a stint in the military, Dr. Hume (figure 29) was recruited in 1949 to direct the orthopedic service at John A. Andrew Memorial Hospital, Tuskegee University, Alabama.

Dr. John W. Chenault[55] (figure 30) was granted a leave of absence to pursue advanced studies that would eventually qualify him to become certified by the American Board of Orthopedic Surgery, leaving his position open for Dr. Hume. Chenault's certification, which allowed him to direct the polio facility, was mandated by the National Foundation for Infantile Paralysis (NFIP), and in 1953 he became the third black diplomate of the American Board of Orthopedic Surgery.[56]

In 1948, the VA Hospital in Tuskegee established an approved residency program in general surgery. The subspecialties of orthopedics, urology, and ophthalmology were necessary elements in the general surgical program. Dr. Hume joined the VA Hospital staff as chief of orthopedics in 1950[57] and continued to serve the Infantile Paralysis Unit with Dr. Chenault until 1955, when the latter entered into private practice in Florida. The surgical residents from the VA

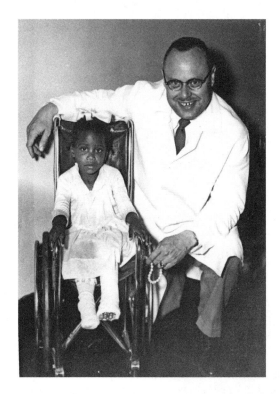

Figure 29. John F. Hume
with a young polio patient.
(Courtesy of the Tuskegee
University Archives)

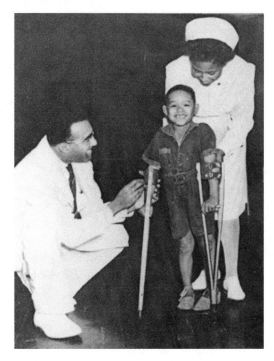

Figure 30. John W. Chenault
and a nurse attending
a young polio patient.
(Courtesy of the Tuskegee
University Archives)

Hospital rotated through the orthopedic service[58] of the John A. Andrew Memorial Hospital, which exposed them also to the case studies of the Crippled Children Service and Polio Unit. Rotations at the John A. Andrew Memorial Hospital allowed them to assist in surgery as well as in the clinics, thus receiving a diversified experience in orthopedic conditions. By 1971, approximately forty residents and interns and several hundred nurses had received training in the hospital and the School of Nursing at Tuskegee University.[59]

Nursing Education

Discrimination toward black nursing students followed much the same pattern as it had against black medical students. As of October 15, 1962, 165 of the 1,128 nursing schools in the United States still did not admit black people, and until 1962 white schools in Alabama and South Carolina had never admitted a black student. Conversely, Tuskegee University's nursing program (figure 31), begun in 1891, was designed, planned, and modeled on black nursing programs at Spelman College in Atlanta and Dixie Hospital in Hampton, Virginia. Furthermore, Tuskegee's program ranged from patient care to household chores and was under the supervision of the JAAMH.[60]

The Tuskegee program was designed for culturally deprived students, mainly from rural areas. In addition to a liberal arts education, it provided clinical nursing experiences, in which students rotated through area hospitals for training while also aiding in meeting the needs of a depressed nursing staff. By 1921, approximately one hundred and forty graduate nurses had received training at Tuskegee and were working all over the country. They were primarily involved in public health nursing, private practices, and working at smaller institutions. A 1918 graduate of the Nursing School, Miss Bessie Hawes, exemplifies the importance these young women felt about their profession. Writing of her experience during the great influenza epidemic of 1919, she related:

> I shall tell you of an experience of which I am very proud. Eight miles from Talladega, Alabama, in the backwoods, a colored family of ten was in bed dying for the want of attention. No one would come near. I was asked by the health officer if I would go. I was glad of the opportunity. As I entered the little country cabin I found the mother dead in bed, the father and the remainder of the family running temperatures of 102 and 104. Some had influenza and others had pneumonia. No relatives or friends would come near. I saw at a glance that I had much work to do. I rolled up my sleeves, killed chickens, and began to cook. I forgot I was not a cook. I only thought of saving lives. I milked the cow, gave medicine, and did everything I could to help conditions. I worked day and

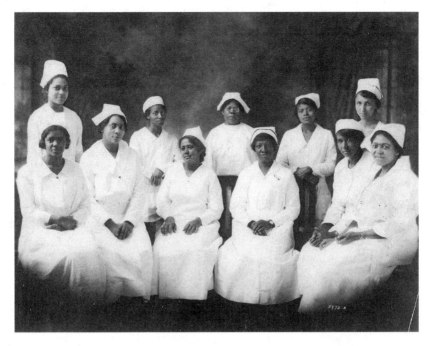

Figure 31. Tuskegee Hospital nurses, c. 1910. (Courtesy of the Tuskegee University Archives)

night trying to save them for seven days. I had no place to sleep. I didn't realize how tired I was until I got home. I sat up at night alone, and one night with a corpse in the house. The doctor lived about twenty miles away and came every other day. He thought I was very brave but I didn't realize 'til it was all over, just how brave I had been. I did, however, feel very happy when they were all out of danger. I only wish I could have reached them earlier and had been able to do something for the poor mother.[61]

The hospital at Tuskegee found yet another way to provide health care for the surrounding communities. Due to its involvement in extension programs, a four-month course of intensive training in midwifery[62] (figure 32) was instituted in an attempt to comply with a 1918 Alabama state law. The legislation required all midwives, white and black, to pass an examination and register with the State Board of Health.[63] Furthermore, the first school in which graduate nurses received specialized training in midwifery opened in September 1941. Sponsored by the Julius Rosenwald Fund, the Alabama State Department of Health, the Children's Bureau, and Tuskegee University, the school owed its in-

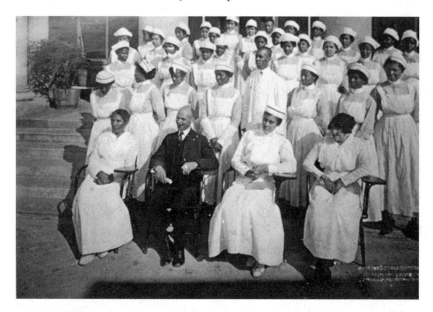

Figure 32. Dr. John A. Kenney and Tuskegee midwives, c. 1920. (Courtesy of the Tuskegee University Archives)

ception to M. O. Bousefield, a specialist in Negro Health at the Julius Rosenwald Foundation. Following a six-month course, trainees received certificates from the Nurses Training Department of Tuskegee University.[64]

By 1921, the hospital also operated a social hygiene program under the US Interdepartmental Social-Hygiene Board. The program's purpose was to provide improvement in the health and physical development of Tuskegee University's students. Significantly, the program included two physical examinations per year, as well as physical education classes with discussions on venereal disease and hygiene. As part of the program, personal interviews with medical instructors were offered to all students, thereby ensuring they had access to any personal health questions.[65]

In 1944, Dr. Lillian Harvey (1912–1994) (figure 33) was recruited by Frederick D. Patterson, president of Tuskegee University, following her graduation from Columbia University, to come to Tuskegee to be in charge of nursing education. Harvey immediately sought to upgrade the curriculum from a three-year certificate program to the first nursing baccalaureate degree program in the state.[66]

At the time Harvey began her work at Tuskegee, registered nurse was not considered to be a high-prestige position in society. In a personal interview with Harvey (later known as Dean Harvey),[67] she revealed that nurses were considered as almost glorified maids. Many of their duties (including bath-

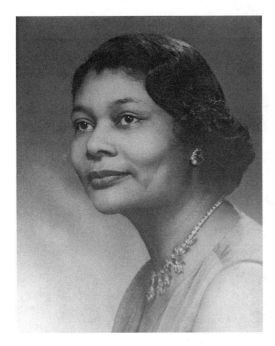

Figure 33. Dr. Lillian Harvey, who established nursing as a baccalaureate program at Tuskegee. (Courtesy of the Tuskegee University Archives)

ing male patients and the disposal of excrement) were considered unfit for a woman of quality.[68] In fact, Alabama forbade white nurses from touching black patients.[69] Therefore, the nursing program had not only to conquer racism and segregation, but also the negative stignas associated with black nurses. Harvey immediately reconstructed the nursing program, recruiting both students and instructors of the highest caliber. This led to Tuskegee becoming one of the outstanding black nursing schools in the country and, in 1947, becoming the first program in Alabama to offer a baccalaureate degree in nursing—not just first for black students, but for anyone.

The program had no individual classroom building;[70] classes were held in the John A. Andrew Memorial Hospital wherever there was a free room there. Most nursing students lived in James Hall, while hired nurses at the hospital lived at the Nurses Home (later known as Lillian Harvey Hall).[71]

Since black nurses were barred from white segregated hospitals and clinics, Harvey set about finding new clinical training sites in order to make certain Tuskegee's student nurses received the highest-quality training for a competitive, mostly white job market. Furthermore, she arranged to have student nurses sent to prestigious institutions such as the Centers for Disease Control in Atlanta, Columbia Hospital in New York City, the Yale School of Medicine and New Haven Hospital, and Massachusetts General Hospital.[72] She set up a curriculum of nurse instructors and hospital staff that was responsible for

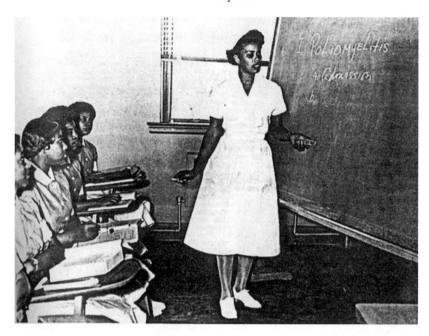

Figure 34. Nursing students learning polio techniques. (Courtesy of the Tuskegee University Archives)

student demonstrations and training. At various stages of their education, lead physician Dr. Chenault and other hospital staff doctors provided important hands-on experiences for the students. Additionally, the veterinary school had many specialists in basic areas such as biology and virology who taught nursing students as well as their own.[73]

Furthermore, the program taught students how to lift and move patients properly and safely, thereby minimizing injury to both the nurse and the patient, as many patients were bedridden and had to be manipulated and moved around several times a day. This instruction was critically important at the newly established Infantile Paralysis wing of the hospital.[74] Once the wing was completed in 1941 and patients began to arrive, it was recognized that this technique was important, especially because all the patients were children and required long-term care. The nursing curriculum was then expanded with a teaching unit developed to specifically deal with the moving and positioning of polio patients (figure 34).

In an interview, Dean Harvey noted that nurses at John A. Andrew Memorial Hospital were very dedicated and employed there for many years. The nurses worked well with each other. They understood and provided support for the student nurses as they dealt with the special frustrations and needs of young polio patients.[75] Due to problems particular to the Infantile Paralysis wing, nursing students had opportunities to observe interdepartmental cooperation, providing them with the best possible training experiences.

Liaison with National Foundation for Infantile Paralysis

Unfortunately, while JAAMH was an excellent health-care facility for black patients, a poliomyelitis (polio) epidemic swept through the South in 1936, crippling black children and adults, thereby overwhelming the hospital's ability to provide appropriate, specialized treatment. The institutions capable of effectively treating poliomyelitis were either too far away to permit travel for poor rural black people or were only open to white patients. Therefore, black polio patients really had nowhere to turn for critically needed care.

The John A. Andrew Clinic Society, which arose out of the actual hospital Clinic, was an important factor leading to the establishment, in 1939, of a polio center attached to the John A. Andrew Memorial Hospital. Specific to the society's meetings were demonstrations, booths, and films from the National Foundation for Infantile Paralysis (NFIP). The information provided by the NFIP helped propel the idea for a facility specifically intended to help black polio patients. Additionally, the need for such a facility arose from the efforts of black doctors such as Dr. John W. Chenault, who witnessed the devastation of the disease on black polio patients within the pediatric clinic of the hospital while attending the Clinic in 1936.

Chenault, who was a mentee of pediatrician Dr. Tom Campbell Jr., son of T. M. Campbell, identified the critical need for specialized long-term care for recovery. Because it was assumed within the white medical community that black people could not contract polio, the hospital was ill-prepared to provide necessary treatment protocols. Naomi Rogers, writing in her groundbreaking article "Race and the Politics of Polio: Warm Springs, Tuskegee, and the March of Dimes," emphatically states:

> It was true that few Black polio victims were reported during the 1920s and 1930s, even with the growing number of epidemics in the Northeast and Midwest. And in the South, where the majority of Black Americans lived until after World War II, there were few outbreaks of polio at all. Nonetheless, leaders of the Black medical profession argued that too many Black polio cases were missed as the result of medical racism and neglect: families had limited access to doctors and hospitals, and inadequately trained Black health professionals were unable to diagnose polio's ambiguous early symptoms. "I firmly believe," Black orthopedist John Watson Chenault asserted, that the statistics used to argue for a lower

incidence of disease among Blacks "are due to the notoriously poor treatment facilities available for Negroes and[,] as much as I hate to admit it, the failure of so many of our men to recognize the disease."[76]

Chenault's subsequent work rallied national attention to the plight of black children with polio who had no facilities for treatment. There were treatment facilities for white patients, but due to segregation there were none for black ones. Furthermore, the Clinic later reached many other black practitioners who were on the front lines of the fight against polio, providing them with up-to-date diagnostic and treatment information. Regarding the Clinic and preparatory to the Infantile Paralysis Center, Dr. John A. Kenney wrote:

> It has been no simple task in this section to induce people to come to the hospital for treatment, because, isolated as they are, they have inherited the very common and very erroneous idea that a hospital is the last resort in case of sickness. [It] has required patience, perseverance, and education gradually to change this idea. [In] the early days, in our smaller building, it was rather difficult to make the Tuskegee students feel at home in the hospital, and the admission of an outside patient from the surrounding communities was a rarity . . . every cured patient who leaves the hospital satisfied is a walking advertisement. . . . [It] is not a rare thing now for parents in our immediate communities to entrust their ailing children promptly to our care; occasionally some parent further away in the country will do likewise. [T]his means we have made a long stride from the beginning; it has taken much time to do it.[77]

The liaison between Tuskegee University and the NFIP resulted in many valuable educational experiences for the Tuskegee staff and students, as well as the surrounding community. Because in the 1930s the black medical community was unaware of polio in black children,[78] they lacked the skills to diagnose the disease and were incapable of providing specific treatment protocols. Therefore, the NFIP provided continuing education programs for Black physicians. This was accomplished when "An institute sponsored by the Georgia State chapter of the National Foundation was held at the center in June of 1944. Part of the teaching staff of the Georgia Warm Springs Foundation, first and oldest polio center located 90 miles from Tuskegee, participated. Six physicians, sixteen public health nurses, six institutional nurses and ten private nurses attended."[79] Many black health professionals received training under NFIP grants. Dr. John W. Chenault received his internship for orthopedic board certification. Nurse Warrena A. Turpin, who was in charge of the Infantile Paralysis unit's nursing service from 1941 until 1948, received continuing education in polio treatment. Due to the NFIP's commitment, physical therapists were encouraged to take advantage of these opportunities.

The NFIP also provided funds for continued education of staff members in order to keep current their knowledge in treatment modalities. Such a group from the Tuskegee Infantile Paralysis Center attended a five-day course in Houston, Texas, at the Southeastern Respiratory Center following the recommendation of Dr. Kenneth Landauer of the NFIP. The Tuskegee group gained valuable experience and were able to set up referrals to the Texas Center. Other educational activities were made possible as an outgrowth of the cooperation between Tuskegee University and the NFIP. Local and regional meetings, conferences, and seminars sponsored by the NFIP were frequently held in Tuskegee. Events held in nearby Montgomery usually featured a trip to the polio treatment center at Tuskegee and stimulated subsequent discussions of the work being done there.[80] Such activity made the work at Tuskegee more visible to the academic and medical community at large.

State of Alabama personnel often visited the Infantile Paralysis Center at Tuskegee. Among those visiting were Mrs. Winningham, superintendent, and R. B. Bagley, assistant director, both of the State Crippled Children's Services, and Frank Jenkins and Homer Jacobs of the Vocational Rehabilitation Department. Many others visited due to the uniqueness of the medical treatment, care, and education exhibited by the well-trained black medical professionals in a predominately black community. This news came to the attention of important black officials throughout the world (such as President William V. S. Tubman of Liberia) who, after visiting the center, would return to their countries and build similar schools.[81]

Substandard health care among black Alabamians and southerners had been a source of great concern, prompting a need for black health-care professionals trained for a variety of conditions. Continuing in the spirit of Booker T. Washington and Robert Moton, Tuskegee University President F. D. Patterson sought to have Tuskegee at the center of health care among black citizens within the state of Alabama and throughout the South. This goal was accomplished by circumventing institutional racism and segregation and working together with white people on a variety of health-care issues. Through the John A. Andrew Clinic, the clinical society, the nursing school, the hospital, and the VA Hospital, Tuskegee University rose to prominence as a place where black and white health-care professionals could work together as colleagues. Regarding this, Patterson wrote: "The John A. Andrew Society has for years served as a nation-wide clinic for Negro physicians and has proven especially valuable to those of the South."[82] Thus was laid the foundation for development of a research laboratory on the campus of Tuskegee University, which would prove instrumental in the NFIP's program to eradicate polio.

3
The National Foundation
for Infantile Paralysis and the
Carver Research Foundation

When the announcement came that the polio vaccine developed by the University of Pittsburgh research team was "safe, effective, and potent," it was no accident that it occurred on April 12, 1955, the 10th anniversary of FDR's death. FDR's leadership in the establishment of the Georgia Warm Springs Foundation, the National Foundation for Infantile Paralysis, and the March of Dimes had finally triumphed over the disease he himself had struggled with for more than half his adult life.

—Mark A. Nordenberg, *Defeat of an Enemy*

Under his skillful massage, with the aid of the oil, he had rubbed away many pains and aches, had restored and strengthened muscles. But his boy had infantile paralysis. Carver made no promises, but set to work.

—Shirley Graham and George D. Lipscomb,
Dr. George Washington Carver, Scientist

The association between the March of Dimes and Tuskegee University proved to be very interesting. The problem of polio affected both white and black people, and yet each took different paths in seeking treatment and, eventually, prevention. A variety of venues had, early on, devoted and developed medical methods and resources for white patients. Hospitals provided treatment throughout the nation but primarily for white patients only. Black patients also sought medical treatment wherever they could and looked to their own scientists for aid. As early as 1928, George Washington Carver at Tuskegee had been focused on helping those suffering from the effects of polio and, with the support of the Tuskegee administration, worked closely with the John A. Andrew Memorial Hospital on campus. All these various paths toward treatment converged in an outcome that affected millions.

The National Foundation for Infantile Paralysis

The background for Tuskegee's continued work in health care during the time of Frederick D. Patterson and beyond is rooted in the relationship between President Franklin D. Roosevelt (1882–1945), the NFIP, and the university. The

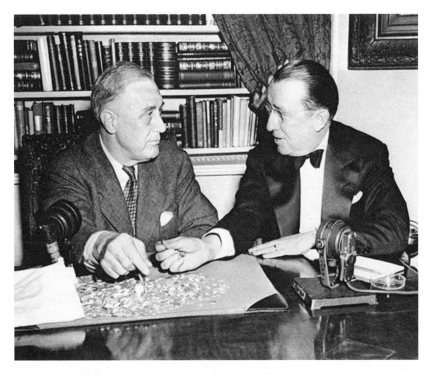

Figure 35. President Franklin D. Roosevelt and Basil O'Connor, FDR's law partner and a cofounder of the National Foundation for Infantile Paralysis. (Courtesy of the Tuskegee University Archives)

bond that developed out of this relationship would propel Tuskegee into an important role in meeting the goals and objectives of the NFIP. Significantly, the role Tuskegee occupied would prove to be substantial beyond the eradication of polio.

The NFIP was founded January 3, 1938, by Roosevelt and his former law partner Basil O'Connor (1892–1972) (figure 35), who was a member and chairman of the Tuskegee University Board of Trustees from 1943 to 1968. The not-for-profit NFIP, today called the March of Dimes, revolutionized fund-raising and the perception of polio in America. They used a variety of techniques including "poster children" and the "march of dimes" campaign, in which they mobilized the public to raise hundreds of millions of dollars to create "the largest research and rehabilitation network in the history of medicine."[1] This allowed them to refrain from relying on a few benefactors who may or may not contribute to their cause. The efforts to find an effective treatment for polio resulted not only in changes to the methodologies of fund-raising, but also led to changes in government regulations.

Prior to the 1962 Kefauver-Harris Amendments, governmental regulation of drug testing and trials were nonexistent. Therefore, the protocols for testing of drugs specific to the prevention of polio focused on the need for more stringent government licensing and testing of drugs prior to their release. This further changed manufacturers' liabilities for releasing drugs that may have proven unsafe or ineffective.

Due to President Roosevelt's own battle with the disease, by 1937 he was convinced polio could only be eradicated through a dedicated course of scientific research and public education. The act of establishing the NFIP as an organization promoted his agenda while going far beyond his own expectations. Dr. Saul Benison, a researcher and specialist in the history of medicine and science, confirmed: "At a time when deadly assault had already been launched against the human spirit and life itself through war in Europe, the new Foundation stood as an affirmation of the value of conserving human life and dignity. Ordinary people everywhere recognized the quality and quietly and emphatically made its cause their own."[2]

Poliomyelitis, commonly called polio or infantile paralysis (because it primarily affects children), is not a modern disease. Evidence suggests the ancient Egyptians suffered from the disease.[3] Although poliomyelitis has existed since before the pre-Christian era, the first recorded cases appeared in the United States, particularly Louisiana, in 1841. Although there were probably many others, the first recognized US polio epidemic occurred in Vermont in 1894, with 132 total cases of which there were 18 deaths, including several cases in adults.[4] By 1916, "the 20 states that kept records of infectious diseases reported 27,367 cases and 7,179 deaths."[5]

In August 1921, Roosevelt joined his family at his estate on the Canadian island of Campobello, hoping to enjoy some much-needed rest and family fun. He was very tired, not having had a long vacation in many years. Always active and athletic, he looked forward to the water sports he so greatly enjoyed. On August 10, he swam in the cold waters of Passamaquoddy Bay, and by the next morning, he awoke to symptoms of fever, weakness, and paralysis in his extremities. During the next few days, the paralysis worsened. Initially, he was misdiagnosed with a blood clot, but later it was determined he had polio. He continued to exercise and recover at home, but it was a year later, in September 1922, before Roosevelt returned to work.[6] The impact of a public figure, who was later elected president of the United States, regardless of his partial paralysis, cannot be underestimated. This was a tremendous force in the development of state-of-the-art treatment plans and finding a cure for one of the most dreaded diseases of all times. Because he was a nationally known figure who had almost endless contacts at his fingertips, he was able to design and promote an agenda that would, in the end, successfully accomplish a feat the magnitude of which could probably never happen again: the capability to eradicate polio.

In the years that followed 1921, Roosevelt learned all he could about the disease affecting his body, including various treatment plans, equipment, and cures, both conventional and unconventional. In 1924, he heard about a place where there might be a cure. In the small, southern community of Warm Springs, Georgia, there was a spring pouring warm water into an outside pool. After swimming in the pool's waters and enjoying the moderate seasons, he was convinced he could walk better and felt more improved than in other place he had visited.

In 1926, he bought the property for "nearly $200,000 (roughly two-thirds of his private fortune)," and incorporated it under the name of Meriwether Reserve.[7] At the time, Roosevelt envisioned the facility for both polio patients and able-bodied vacationers, the income from the latter to support the former.[8] Upon advice from some friends, he decided in 1927 to make Warm Springs a therapeutic facility focusing on the strengthening of muscle movement in polio patients. The new endeavor was renamed the Georgia Warm Springs Foundation. A hospital was constructed that would provide physical therapy and rehabilitation for polio victims. The location later included facilities for corrective surgery, using the latest techniques for repairing muscles that polio had permanently contracted. As governor of the state of New York, Roosevelt began to emphasize that "money spent to make cripples wage-earners would 'come back many times through their increased productiveness.'"[9] This resulted in a program at Warm Springs that addressed the needs of crippled adults and children, wherever they resided.

When Roosevelt reentered politics in 1928, he appointed Basil O'Connor as director of the Warm Springs Foundation. Within the year, O'Connor had hired Keith Morgan,[10] a successful insurance salesman, to be the public relations spokesman. Morgan was responsible for "selling the concept of Warm Springs to wealthy people."[11] Unfortunately, donations substantially declined due to the stock market crash and subsequent Depression.[12] Limited funds prohibited growth, and by 1932, only $30,000 had been raised to cover expenses. This meant new patients were not admitted to the facility. David Oshinsky writes in the book *Polio: An American Story*, "All of a sudden there were fewer rich people with a lot less to give. . . . With the Depression, Warm Springs almost went under. . . . There was no money to pay bills."[13]

Morgan appealed to his friend Carl Byoir[14] for help in fund-raising and public relations. During a brainstorming session, Byoir suggested that the president's birthday could be used to organize annual parties/balls all across the country as a way to raise funds to support the Warm Springs program. Out of this idea arose the National Committee for Birthday Balls,[15] which launched celebrations on January 29, 1934, in which approximately 6,000 balls were held; with the most lavish at the Waldorf-Astoria in New York City. Later, the committee's name was changed to the President's Birthday Ball Commission for Infantile Paralysis Research so funds could be awarded to medical researchers seeking a cure for polio.[16]

Due to a severe recession in 1937 and the limited distribution of funds from the balls, revenues began to decline and the issue of polio treatment and research became a political issue for Roosevelt. A new strategy was needed to depoliticize the polio crusade. "In 1938, Roosevelt announced the formation of a nonpartisan group to be called the National Foundation for Infantile Paralysis. Its major aims, he said, were to find a cure for polio while providing the best treatment for those already afflicted."[17] Roosevelt's old friend and confidant Basil O'Connor was appointed as the new foundation's president. The institution would take the focus of the funding specifically away from the Warm Springs Foundation, making it a truly national endeavor, making it possible for polio patients around the country to benefit from funding through research and treatment in their own regions.[18]

The NFIP became official on January 3, 1938. The new organization was a consolidation of the earlier institutions with emphasis on utilizing fund-raising as a means to finance patient care, medical research, and "professional education programs to augment patient care."[19] Author Theo Lippman noted, "the new foundation soon proved to be one of the most imaginative fund-raising enterprises the world of cheerful giving had ever seen or ever would see."[20] Indeed, it "became the 'gold standard' for private charities, the largest voluntary health organization of all times, its success in raising money, generating publicity, caring for patients, and sponsoring medical research would serve to redefine the role—and the methods—of private philanthropy in the United States."[21]

As part of his strategy to reach more people, O'Connor enlisted Hollywood movie stars, entertainers, and vaudeville veterans. These gladly accepted the request, because they knew it would provide them with important publicity. During a strategy session, actor Eddie Cantor (1892–1964) invented and began using on his live radio show the slogan "March of Dimes" in order to solicit contributions.[22] This campaign involved asking for dimes to be sent to the White House specifically for use by the NFIP. Shortly thereafter, little cards were developed that held ten dimes each (figure 36). The idea was that "everybody could give a dime." This promotion raised millions of dollars for the foundation. The theme was publicized in conjunction with the President's Birthday Balls, with celebrities using their popularity to make special appeals over the radio and in theaters.

In 1942, the NFIP adopted the idea of a "poster child," which significantly added to the publicity package.[23] The poster child campaign put a face on polio. Often children were chosen for the posters based on the severity of their dis-

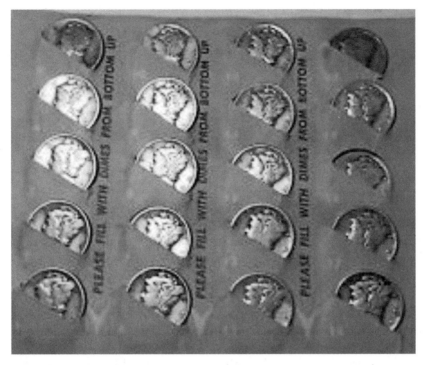

Figure 36. March of Dimes card filled with Liberty Head dimes. (Courtesy of the Tuskegee University Archives)

ability. In 1949, stage siren Helen Hayes (1900–1993) lost her daughter, Mary MacArthur, to polio, and became devoted to seeking a cure. She promoted the March of Dimes as the National Mothers March Chairwoman (1951–1961).[24]

Both the National Mothers March and the poster child campaign played upon the sympathies of families throughout the nation. Women, specifically mothers, canvassed neighborhoods from house to house for donations, which led to the Mothers' March that began in 1950. Officially called the "Mothers' March on Polio," the movement originated in Phoenix, Arizona, with the signature "leave the front porch light on," indicating the homeowners' willingness to make a donation. Although their focus has somewhat changed, both of these campaigns continue today, in one form or another, with the NFIP.[25]

Although the NFIP had expanded its emphasis nationally, the building effort at Warm Springs continued to increase. The hospital, a school, and an occupational therapy building were built in 1939, followed by a chapel, dorms, and a brace shop. Concurrent to the building expansion, the staff became more skilled and specialized.[26] The primary mission of the NFIP was to "lead, direct and unify the fight" against polio.[27] So, as part of their national program, the

NFIP put into action, at Warm Springs and elsewhere, the response to their mission by paying "all expenses and all patient care costs."[28]

Basil O'Connor continued to serve as president of the NFIP from 1938 to 1972. An unsung hero, much of his work during his affiliation was behind the scenes. No doubt, after 1950, he was further driven by the fact that his daughter, Bettyann, had contracted the very disease that he had worked so hard to eradicate.[29] David Rose, archivist at the March of Dimes, noted that O'Connor's greatest accomplishment was "the leadership of the fundraising crusade, the March of Dimes, based on the philanthropy of common people and the co-ordination of a massive medical research effort that led to the creation of the Salk vaccine."[30] Dr. Luther H. Foster (1900–1981), president of Tuskegee University (1953–1981), eulogized Tuskegee Board of Trustee member[31] O'Connor, in 1972, saying, "Basil O'Connor knew how to frame a philosophy for action. When equal employment opportunity was but a twinkle on the horizon, he took steps to make this thesis real in the March of Dimes and The National Foundation. In the early days of attack on polio, Basil O'Connor joined with Tuskegee associates to make sure there was at least one center in the country where black patients could have access to polio treatment in a setting of human dignity and with high professional care."[32] Dr. Melvin Glasser, Chairman of the National Foundation's Executive Board of Trustees, at the same service, said, "Basil O'Connor said repeatedly, 'I don't want to be remembered as the best voluntary agency fund raiser this country ever had.' But he was. Brilliant administrator, effective organizer, inspired leader, he attracted to him and the causes for which he fought, able staff and a dedicated army of volunteers. . . . They were part of a new social institution he created—the voluntary health agency, national in character, supported by huge numbers of very small gifts."[33] No doubt, O'Connor left a lasting legacy that few have recognized or publicized. One can but wonder how successful the NFIP would have been without this stalwart leader.

After implementing a means of treating victims of infantile paralysis, the first of the NFIP's two main goals, they now focused on the search for an effective vaccine. This emphasis on a preventative was due to the increased number of polio cases that had begun to rise, both in numbers and severity, from 2000 cases in 1940, to 58,000 cases in 1952 (including both white and black people). Most of these cases were children; thus, the search became more critical.[34] This did not go unnoticed by members of the black community and certainly not by Tuskegee University.

The George Washington Carver Research Foundation

Because of O'Connor's relationship with Tuskegee and the George Washington Carver Research Foundation (GWCRF), the NFIP also later utilized black scientists in the search for aprevention for polio. Two questions arise: How were these scientists prepared for such an undertaking? Why did O'Connor and the NFIP become so convinced these scientists could accomplish such a feat? The answers to both questions begins with the founding of the GWCRF by George Washington Carver himself.[35]

Amidst the angst of segregation, Carver established the GWCRF to provide funding for education and research opportunities for deserving young black students. During this time, black academics were often excluded by white academics, without being afforded respect for their scholarship or equality in academe. Carver's philosophy was not one of exclusion but of development. He sought ways to integrate agriculture and medicine in a holistic method similar to those in use today. His scientific work was broad and included a wide variety of interests, including plant diseases, bacteriology, medicinal herbs, dietary supplements, and the use of agricultural products in industry.[36] This was exemplified in his work with polio patients.

Early on, Carver developed a deep interest in working with the medicinal properties of herbs and oils that he had incorporated as a "rubber for the athletic teams at Ames, Iowa."[37] Later, after several experiments, as early as 1928, Carver began to believe his formula for a peanut oil rubbing emulsion and his massaging regimen would benefit those suffering from the effects of polio. Writing in 1934 to Dr. Eugene Dibble,[38] who was then employed as medical director at the John A. Andrew Memorial Hospital in Tuskegee, Carver described his method of using the emulsion on polio patients: "The muscles needing it most should be singled out and massaged daily. Great care should be taken in the gentleness and thoroughness with which it is done. Five or six drops only of this oil should be used at a time, massaged until every trace has disappeared. Repeat this as long as the skin and weak muscles will take it up, then stop until the next day."[39] He goes on to note, "if done thoroughly and properly the skin and muscles should become super saturated in nine days."[40]

Carver was convinced of the efficacy of his ointment, and he was not the only one. At one point in 1934, he said "my infantile paralysis cases are keeping me almost more than busy. I have nearly 40 patients that I am giving my personal attention."[41] Carver cautioned he was not a physician and would often advise "his patients" to seek proper medical care (figure 37).[42] There were indeed many success stories. Typical correspondence regarding his suggested procedures and emulsions include comments stating, "His leg is slowly improving" and "he is improving most satisfactory." At one point in 1935, Carver wrote to his longtime friend Dr. M. L. Ross, of Topeka, Kansas, "one of my worst patients has taken off both of his leg braces and is using his crutches only and walking better than he has in 22 years."[43] This prompted a variety of newspaper accounts that, no doubt, accelerated his fame and abilities throughout the nation and abroad (figure 38).[44]

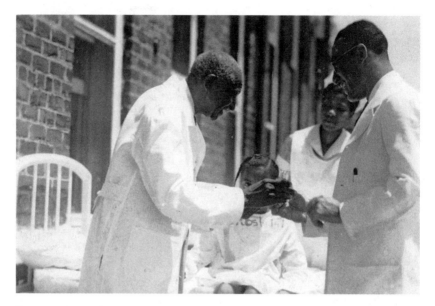

Figure 37. Carver with a young patient and hospital staff. (Courtesy of the Tuskegee University Archives)

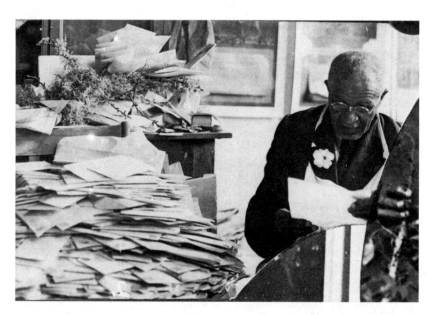

Figure 38. Carver reading his voluminous correspondence. (Courtesy of the Tuskegee University Archives)

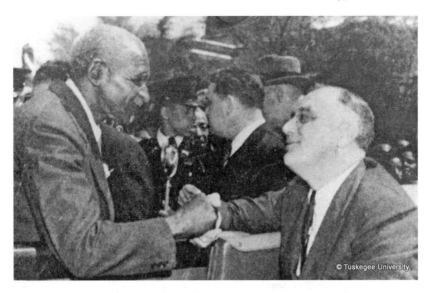

© Tuskegee University

Figure 39. Carver and Roosevelt meeting on Tuskegee's campus, March 1939. (Courtesy of the Tuskegee University Archives)

In 1938, Carver sent President Roosevelt a sample of his peanut oil. Although not a public gesture, he was seeking to secure support for his treatment protocol (figure 39).[45] The president later responded, "I do use peanut oil from time to time and I am sure that it helps."[46]

Many within the medical profession sought to discredit Carver concerning the peanut oil emulsion and the procedures used to apply it. These scientists felt that since the peanut oil probably did not have any medical advantage, it was of a minimal help at best and spurious at worst.[47] Furthermore, the American Medical Association felt Carver was improperly portraying himself as a medical doctor. Both were ignorant of his true intentions. The success of "his patients" was due to two important factors: the peanut oil provided an unguent coupled with brisk massaging to heat the muscles. The heat from the procedures utilized by Carver helped to increase blood flow to the affected area. This increased flow, in turn, helped to reduce muscle spasms by increasing the amount of oxygen reaching the injured tissue. This was the forerunner of the work undertaken by "the later and more famous Sister Kenny."[48] Significantly, Carver did not receive any financial benefit from this work, and his labors were directed toward both black and white patients.

There were some physicians who did not agree with the poor assessment of Carver and his work. In May 1935, Carver received on a prescription note a request from Dr. J. F. Fargason, a white doctor of East Tallassee, Alabama, to see a Mr. Fields, a white man, who had been diagnosed with cancer. Apparently, he was "desirous of your seeing him and making any suggestions that you may see fit."[49] In a letter to Dr. L. C. Fischer, Carver wrote: "You thrill me when you say that if possible you will come down and look into the work that I am doing on Infantile Paralysis."[50] Fischer later responded, "As soon as I can spare the time am going to write you a few days ahead of a visit and see if it is possible to have several of your patients at the institute, let us talk with and examine them. Your work may mean a great deal to sufferers. I am prepared to believe this when I have seen the wonderful things you have done with the work that has been your life's interest."[51] Carver's work not only excited himself and his patients but also those of his colleagues that were open to the work of others who were not trained/educated physicians.

Carver's career at Tuskegee began in 1896 and ended with his death in January 1943, a total of 47 years, yet his legacy would continue on in the work done by those who followed him at Tuskegee. Author Ethel Edwards would later write, "With the crippled children, and to a lesser degree with youthful ball players and tense adults, God worked through him to relieve suffering humanity."[52]

The importance of Carver's work and legacy cannot be overemphasized. His vision to provide an outlet for black scientific discovery in an environment free from institutional racism and segregation came to fruition in the establishment of the George Washington Carver Research Foundation. The foundation's beginnings are far from shadowy or incomplete. Carver's thrift and altruistic desire to be of service to humanity allowed him to amass a considerable sum at that time, in spite of the fact that his salary varied little throughout his entire tenure.

As he aged and his health began to fail, his concern over what to do with his savings became more acute. Moreover, he wanted to "preserve and continue his techniques of research, his methods of finding new uses for native materials and his scientific approach to the problem of agriculture and industry."[53] In order to facilitate this, Carver sought to maintain his products, paintings, laces, woodcarvings, and bulletins into a collection for the benefit of all. His assistant, Austin Curtis,[54] came up with the idea to set up a foundation to encourage creative research and preserve each of Carver's collections.[55]

During the 1936–1937 school year, Carver's fortieth year at Tuskegee, the administration planned a celebration to coincide with commencement that would pay tribute to his many accomplishments. The celebration included many of his collections that had been retrieved from various places on campus and arranged by Curtis. The displays were an immediate hit with students, faculty, staff, and alumni, resulting in the Tuskegee University Board of Trustees providing the collections with a permanent home. In 1941, the Carver Museum (figure 40)

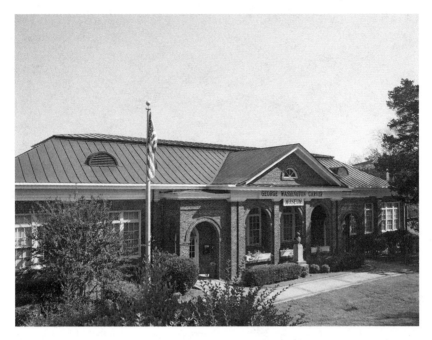

Figure 40. The Carver Museum. (Courtesy of the Tuskegee University Archives)

was opened in the old laundry building, which stood near Dorothy Hall (now the Kellogg Conference Center) on the Tuskegee University campus. The displays were placed on the first floor, and as a further gesture of admiration, Carver and Curtis were allowed to locate their laboratories in the basement.

In the fall of 1937, Carver collapsed and was hospitalized in critical condition; his recuperation took several months. Although he continued to work after that event, he was aware of his frailty and in 1940 bequeathed his entire savings "which, thanks to his fantastic frugality, amounted to some $33,000" to Tuskegee University.[56] Carver decided to make his donation known while he was alive so he could assure it was properly used. Through his efforts, the seed money was put toward the George Washington Carver Foundation.

Established on February 10, 1940, the foundation sought to "provide facilities and a measure of support for young Negroes engaged in advanced scientific research."[57] Upon his death in 1943, Carver willed his entire estate to the university, making his total contribution over $60,000.[58] Per Carver's desires, the foundation was charged with the responsibility of training young people in the scientific approach, all in an attempt to solve the problems of agriculture and industry as they relate to the South. To that end, the GWCRF was made up of the following:

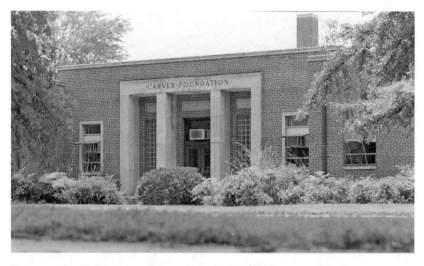

Figure 41. The Carver Research Foundation Building. (Courtesy of the Tuskegee University Archives)

1. The Research Division, which continued the kind of scientific research begun by Carver and through which many capable young people received training in research methods and procedures.
2. The Agricultural Research and Experiment Station, which was concerned with the problems of rural and farm life and the development of new uses for agricultural waste and native materials.
3. The Carver Museum, which preserved and displayed many specimens of the samples and products obtained and produced by Carver. Included in the museum was the Carver Art Collection of paintings and needlework.
4. The director of the foundation was also the director of the Agricultural Research and Experiment Station. Therefore, the Carver Foundation served as a virtual clearinghouse for all research activities at Tuskegee.[59]

Throughout the years, the GWCRF has endeavored to maintain the principles upon which it was founded, and it was under the Research Division that the work on a preventative for polio was conducted.

From 1941 to 1947, the Carver Research Foundation was located in the Carver Museum; then from 1947–1951, it was temporarily housed in the old veterinary hospital located between Campbell Hall and Milbank Hall, which had been built in 1900. Later, utilizing some of the funds left by Carver, a new building was built in 1952 and located adjacent to Armstrong Hall (figure 41). It is from this building that Tuskegee's work with the polio vaccine began.

Carver's legacy of working toward the betterment of mankind through the use of Tuskegee's laboratories would come to fruition. Regarding the work of the GWCRF, Tuskegee faculty member and author Dr. B. D. Mayberry wrote: "For close to 50 years, the Carver Research Foundation was an integral part of Tuskegee University and the campus building so named still serves as a living, operating, and confirmed monument to the contributions of Dr. George Washington Carver in the areas of applied agricultural and basic life science research and education at the university. The Foundation was a product of Dr. Carver's own creativity and foresight. He envisioned it as both a means of the continuation of 'Chemurgy,' his scientific approach to problems in agriculture, and as means of preserving and utilizing his methods and techniques of finding new uses for native materials in the interest of people."[60] Fulfillment of Carver's dream for the GWCRF began in an astonishing manner and scale. All of this was made possible by a unique convergence of circumstance and opportunity for which Tuskegee, against history's long odds, found itself well prepared.

4
The Search for the Vaccine

Everybody in the public health field knows that when you reach the point where you can begin to inoculate an agent into millions of children, your problems have only just begun.
—Laurie Garrett, *Betrayal of Trust*, 139

The timing of Tuskegee's involvement in the search for a cure for polio was not coincidental. Rather, it was the culmination of many years of health-related research and involvement in public outreach, education, and intensive experimental research. Tuskegee became an island of intensive work in agriculture and health care, despite its size, obscure location, and dedication to the teaching of young black men and women during a time of racial segregation. It was of little interest to larger, more fully funded academic institutions. Yet, its involvement with the NFIP would propel Tuskegee to a prominent place in history.

In order to understand the complexities of the relationship between the NFIP, its objective, and Tuskegee, it would no doubt prove helpful to understand the unique terminology used in the medical field as it applies to the work Tuskegee was to provide. This work entailed developing methods to propagate, store, and distribute significant quantities of live cell cultures to be used in the largest single research project ever conducted (which will probably never again be equaled).

The project succeeded at Tuskegee by involving a large group of individuals and institutions seeking a common goal. Their interactions with each other are crucial to understanding how the goal of successfully obtaining a preventative for polio developed.

Immunology: A Primer

It is important to define terms, concepts, and protocols before embarking on a short discussion of immunology. Immunology is the study of the way the human body reacts to a potentially infectious agent.[1] There are specific phases in the research process that must take place before a vaccine can be developed and made available to the public. This process includes important protocols established to test the efficacy[2] and safety of the vaccine. It is important to understand both the details pertinent to viruses and the antibodies formed in the host to fight viral infection, in addition to knowing how a vaccine is made. These details provide a link to poliovirus, the polio vaccine, and the researchers who worked on the vaccine. Likewise, it is especially necessary to gain an appreciation of the time, effort, skill, and expense demanded in order to put all the components together when searching for and developing a new vaccine. In general, it takes about ten very expensive years to bring a new drug to the marketplace,[3] yet in the case of the polio vaccine, the last critical steps were completed in about four years. The dedication of the NFIP researchers was unparalleled. This also speaks to the trust placed by the NFIP in the Tuskegee researchers, as well their abilities to carry out needed protocols and procedures.

In the 1940s and 1950s, immunology and virology were newly emerging specialties. Typically, in the laboratory, bacteria and molds grow on media plates.[4] Although there are other steps involved, a small sample could be put on a slide and viewed under the microscope to determine what strain of bacteria or mold was present. However, a virus will not grow on routine laboratory media. This was a major problem, since a vaccine cannot be produced against a virus until the researchers can determine its composition or structure and how it caused the disease. Like chicken pox, measles, mumps, and warts, poliomyelitis is a viral disease. The virus particle is:

> less than one-millionth of an inch across, contains ribonucleic acid, which determines its nature, and a protein shell that coats the tiny shred of identity, protects it, and guides it in its journey with the living organism to the particular types of cell that can be its host[5] . . . the virus particle springs to life only when it enters a living cell, where it usually multiplies at so mad a pace that it quickly destroys it nurturing chamber. Within minutes, hundreds of newborn viruses explode out through the cell's shattered walls to find new homes, new cells, and new hosts to devastate. The speed and strength of the individual body's immune system determines how far a virus will travel and how much damage it will do before this multiplication is stopped. The complex process may take several weeks; if too many vital cells are destroyed before the immune system marshals its forces, the infected person dies. Those fortunate to survive a viral infection are left with a system of antibodies and memory cells that are primed to stop that particular virus at once, should it ever enter the body again. This triumph of biological memory is known as immunity.[6]

To counteract and neutralize a viral attack, one must have a good titer[7] of the appropriate antibodies that have been made by that individual's body to recognize, attack, and destroy that specific virus. If the patient has never been exposed to a particular virus before, he or she will not have the appropriate level of antibodies and will develop symptoms of whatever disease is caused by that virus. Thus, the idea behind a vaccine becomes one of "tricking" the body into thinking it has been exposed to a virus for the first time. The body will begin to produce the appropriate antibodies, thereby building up a supply that will be available to protect the body (i.e., immunity) from that disease, should the body actually become exposed to the particular virus in the future.

Although a virus (Latin meaning "poisonous slime") that attacked tobacco plants was discovered in 1898 by Martinus Willem Beijernick (1851–1931),[8] he did not realize what he found. In 1935, Wendell Stanley (1904–1971)[9] identified the virus while working at the Rockefeller Institute. Prior to World War I, Alexis Carrel (1873–1944),[10] a French biologist, also working at the Rockefeller Institute, found he could take embryonic cells from the heart of a chicken, put them in a test tube, and add a growth medium for food, and they would stay alive indefinitely.[11] Knowing it was possible to produce viruses in a controlled laboratory setting, a solid piece of the puzzle was identified concerning how viruses grew. Over the next several years, cultivation of many viruses was attempted by this process; some were more successful than others.

The Search for the Polio Vaccine

In 1916, the search for a vaccine against poliomyelitis began.[12] However, there were several unsuccessful starts, particularly in growing the poliovirus. It was not until 1936 that Drs. Albert Sabin[13] and Peter Olitsky (1888–1964) were able to successfully grow the virus using human embryonic nervous tissue in place of the routinely used chicken embryonic heart cells.[14] They had tried other types of human tissues with no success. From that point, the accepted rule, which later proved to be incorrect, was that poliovirus could only be grown in cells collected from tissues obtained from the nervous system.

Dr. John Enders (1897–1985),[15] who had recently come to Boston Children's Hospital from Harvard Medical School, was seeking to develop tissue cultures in order to identify a variety of childhood viral diseases, not including polio. In 1949, he and his assistants, Drs. Tom Weller and Frederick C. Robbins, worked with an assortment of support culture media, called a broth, which usually consisted of nutrient materials.[16] At this point, the broth contained no cells; it was simply a medium for supporting the nutrient needs for the addition of tissue cells specifically dictated by the ongoing research. One day, Weller created too many culture tubes for the experiment he was preparing. Enders suggested he use the leftovers to seed with a poliovirus that had been provided by the NFIP and stored in a freezer. Despite the fact that the culture medium used by Enders's laboratory contained no nervous system tissue cells, the poliovirus proliferated. With this new knowledge, Enders realized enough poliovirus could be grown to make a vaccine, thus earning them the 1954 Nobel Prize in Physiology and Medicine. During the Nobel Prize Award Ceremony, Professor S. Gard, a member of the staff of professors of the Royal Caroline Institute, noted the prize was given to the doctors based upon their "discovery of the capacity of the poliomyelitis virus to grow in test-tube cultures of various tissues" thereby "giving the virologists a practicable method for the isolation and study of viruses."[17]

The methods discovered by Enders and his associates provided a low-cost tissue culture beyond what was previously known. It was routinely assumed by researchers that the poliovirus could multiply only in the spinal cords and brains of infected monkeys. However, additional research showed poliovirus attacked only humans, monkeys, and chimpanzees. Research ethics precluded using humans in clinical trials, thus chimpanzees were used due to their close compatibility. The problem was exacerbated in that they were large, rare, and difficult to keep. The cost of using primates was significant, and "this had been a bottleneck in scientific research."[18] Enders's method permitted hundreds of low-cost studies that were carried out simultaneously in test tubes, rather than in live animals.

In 1948, at the same time Enders and company were making their discoveries, four others had determined there were three types of poliovirus that caused poliomyelitis, which they designated as Type I, II, and III. "Since every strain would have to be included in any successful vaccine, the question then became whether there were no more than three."[19] Primary research came through the efforts of Drs. Howard Howe and David Bodian of Johns Hopkins University, and Drs. James Trask and John Paul of Yale. Their laboratories established there were at least three separate strains of poliovirus. However, to prove there were no more than three, the NFIP established the "Virus Typing Program." In order to reduce the chance of error, the NFIP identified four separate laboratories tasked with testing at least one hundred different samples each.[20] Jonas Salk's laboratory was identified as one of the four that would be involved in the testing. Results were compared, and it was confirmed there were only three types.

The typing program lasted from 1949 to 1951 and cost more than $1,200,000.00.[21] The final results proved useful. Type I contained 82 percent of the strains tested, making it the most common form of polio. Type II contained 10 percent and

Type III 8 percent. Type I was the most virulent of the strains. The prevailing thought was poliovirus bypassed the bloodstream upon entrance into the body; therefore the immune system would not be activated to thwart the virus. However, in early 1952, Dr. Dorothy Horstmann of Yale University (along with Bodian) proved the "poliovirus enters the bloodstream for a time during its journey to attack nerves. This meant that antibodies existing in the blood could, if present in sufficient numbers, meet and defeat poliovirus before it could destroy nerves and thus paralyze muscles. Creation of protective antibodies in the blood stream is the function for which vaccines are designed."[22]

In 1936, when the National Foundation began providing funds for polio research, scientists had believed that poliomyelitis was caused by a virus that attacked the cells of the nervous system. It was also understood that about one-half of the victims recovered with no residual paralysis, and most of the cases occurred in young children. Up to that point, all they could do was scientific observation. Gard defines such observation by noting: "At first the virologist had to resort entirely to animal experiments, hoping that inoculation of the test material would produce a typical disease. Instead of studying the virus itself he must be content to observe the animal's reaction to infection and try to deduce therefrom some information on the properties and the nature of viruses. This indirect method is more labor intensive and time consuming, more expensive, and above all less easily interpreted than the bacteriological culture technique."[23]

But this form of data gathering was insufficient to develop more effective forms of preventative treatment. Since they did not know how it was transmitted, they assumed that when the episodes broke out in the summer, they were the results of direct person-to-person contact through airborne means. They worked in crisis mode. They closed pools, canceled Sunday schools and summer camps, and forbade large gatherings, all in an attempt to minimize transmission of the virus. But the question remained: how was the virus actually transmitted?

It was not until the development of the electron microscope[24] that scientists could see the virus and begin studying samples in order to determine where it might have occurred. Researchers established the virus was harbored in sewers and other places where fecal matter might be found. Before this information was revealed and modern sanitation was practiced, children exposed to the virus in small doses began to build up antibodies to protect themselves.[25] When modern sanitation practices were dictated by health-service organizations, however, the link between protection and disease was broken. Doctors instructed parents to clean hands, home, everything. Exposure to the virus was now substantially limited. Unfortunately, the negative impact was that, when young children were exposed to the virus, they had no previously developed antibodies to protect themselves. Thus, incidents of polio rose due to increased sanitization. After twenty years of intense research and development, scientists had finally found some of the answers to their most urgent questions about the nature and behavior of the virus. These answers were critical to developing a vaccine, and Tuskegee University would be instrumental in this endeavor.

Dr. Jonas Salk

After World War II Pittsburgh's steel industries were booming, and the city was black with soot and smoke. It was so bad that one popular description called the city "Hell with the lid taken off."[26] The city's leadership soon decided to change their national image to one of community development and cleanliness. In order to fulfill this vision, the search was on for increased funding. The University of Pittsburgh, then a much smaller institution than it is today, was soon tagged to become a leader in the advanced training of increased numbers of scientists and technical workers who would lead the city boldly into the twenty-first century. As part of this renewed emphasis on high-tech training, the university became the beneficiary of a large sum of money and began recruiting young, bright research scientists for a new program in virus research. In 1947, Dr. Jonas Salk (figure 42) was one of the first to be hired at the University of Pittsburgh as an associate professor of bacteriology and microbiology.[27]

Salk (1914–1995) received his MD in 1939 from New York University, and, following this, he completed a two-year internship at New York's Mount Sinai Hospital.[28] Initially intending to practice medicine, Salk was soon focusing instead solely on research, attending a variety of seminars helping to perfect his research skills. During his internship, Salk worked in the virus research laboratory of Dr. Thomas Francis Jr. (1900–1969).[29] Francis, a physician, virologist, and epidemiologist, was certainly an asset for Salk, helping him meet two important criteria for developing a good reputation in a competitive field: working in a first class laboratory and having a respected mentor who was also a capable fundraiser. Of equal importance, Francis's name at the top of a paper commanded editorial attention in professional journals. Although Salk's name was secondary, this nonetheless allowed him to develop his own reputation. Following Francis's departure from Mount Sinai to the University of Michigan, Salk requested the opportunity to work with him after completion of his internship. Francis capitulated, and Salk went to Ann Arbor in April 1942, where he worked for the next six years on influenza virus research. During this time, he experimented with a variety of techniques to inactivate viruses, helping him further perfect the skills he would later use in his polio research.[30]

Soon, Salk sought his own research program, desiring to become a principal investigator with his own research laboratory, equipment, and staff. He

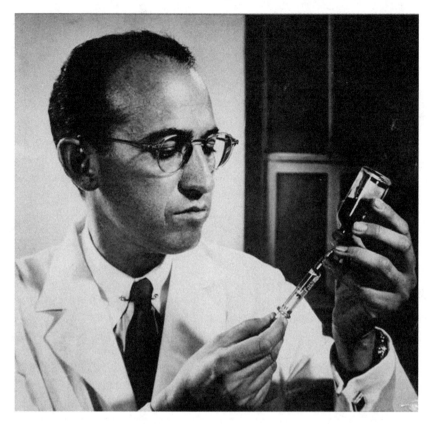

Figure 42. Dr. Jonas Salk. (Courtesy of the March of Dimes Archives, Photo by Yousuf Karsh, 1956)

found his independence at the University of Pittsburgh as a professor in the medical school. At that time, Pittsburgh was not considered one of the top research centers in the country, but the city was on the move and the university was receiving funds. Salk had a vision, and he knew if he could obtain enough outside support, with hard work and determination, he could substantially develop his new laboratory. "At Michigan, Salk had worked in spacious fully equipped quarters, surrounded by a small army of colleagues and staff. At Pittsburgh, he was given two bare rooms in the basement of Municipal Hospital, adjacent to the medical school. His new staff consisted of a single 'secretary-technician.' There were no graduate students to train. His research colleagues, three in number, worked on plant viruses, a subject of little interest to Salk."[31] Salk stayed on, however, seeking another project to increase funding and expand his laboratory. Although outside his field of interest, he agreed to work on the National Foundation for Infantile Paralysis's poliovirus typing project. The NFIP also sought important labs such as those of Drs. David Bodian,[32] Thomas Francis Jr.,[33] and Albert Sabin,[34] but it was Salk's laboratory that did the bulk of the testing.[35] The project was estimated to take approximately three years.

After representatives from John Enders's laboratory announced the discovery that the poliovirus could be grown on medium other than human nervous tissue cells, only Salk recognized he could use these findings to more quickly accomplish his project goals. More than that, though, he could also apply their conclusions to the search for a vaccine. This resulted in a NFIP grant of approximately one million dollars covering 1949 to 1952. Salk had met his goals, and his laboratory grew.

Nature of Viruses and Vaccines

The work of Salk and others revealed a complexity of working with viruses that was, up to this point, little understood. Viruses are very unstable and can mutate, or change, very rapidly. Thus, if a vaccine is made that stimulates antibodies, the virus can mutate in a short while, making those particular antibodies no longer able to recognize or neutralize the newly mutated virus. This means the host is back to square one—with an ineffective vaccine for the new virus.[36]

As already noted, one problem that occurred when working with viruses was the possibility there may be more than one type, or strain, of that particular virus. This meant all types of that virus had to be identified and isolated. In the case of the poliovirus, the researchers suspected there were at least three types of the poliovirus. To be certain, several laboratories were required to test hundreds of samples of poliovirus to see how many types were found. This was critical to the development of a vaccine. An effective vaccine must contain each of the identified types. Finally, the vaccine was tested in humans, with followups that were analyzed in order to determine whether the appropriate antibodies had been produced with each of the types represented. Analysis of the effectiveness of the vaccine was described as follows: "To a tube containing living . . . cells is added some poliovirus mixed with a small sample of blood from a vaccinated youngster. If there are enough antibodies in the child's blood, these antibodies will prevent the virus from killing the cells. In other words, they will protect the cells (thus, the child) against polio."[37] In other words, "If you add virus to the cells, it kills them. Under a microscope you can see this very clearly, because the dead cells simply drop off the walls of the test tube, leaving a blank, or open space."[38] Alternatively, if there are not enough antibodies then "when the poliovirus goes to work it seems to tear huge holes in the tapestry, as the cells shrivel and die (thus, the child is susceptible to polio)."[39] This was a huge undertaking, but Salk was excited to be a part of a project to find a preventative for polio.

Salk's laboratory was one of four chosen by the National Foundation directors for the poliovirus typing program. The other teams were Universities of California, Utah, Kansas, and Pittsburgh. Established researchers involved with polio research at that time were Drs. Albert Sabin at University of Cincinnati, John Enders at Boston Children's Hospital, Thomas M. Rivers at Rockerfeller Institute, Joseph Melnick and John Paul at Yale, Isabel Morgan and David Bodian at Johns Hopkins, Thomas Francis Jr. at University of Michigan, and Hilary Koprowski at Lederle Laboratories (the pharmaceutical division of American Cyanamid in New Jersey). The NFIP's Committee on Research, which was established specifically to search for a preventative for polio, appointed Dr. Harry Weaver as the director.[40] Initially, the committee's scientific advisors were against having someone else in charge. Weaver, however, had worked with the NFIP on several previous projects, and the advisors eventually realized this endeavor required someone in this position.[41] Also, Weaver seemed, early on, to have developed a close relationship with Jonas Salk.[42] While they did not necessarily work together, they shared information they both found useful.

While Salk was working on the typing program, he also received special tips from Weaver about how he could continue to work at the same time on his vaccine. So, when the virus typing program was over in 1952, Salk had enough data to show the NFIP his preparation was safe. Likewise, he now felt it was time to determine the effectiveness of the vaccine to prevent polio.

In a NFIP report published in 1954 titled *Poliomyelitis Vaccine Types 1, 2, and 3*,[43] the Vaccine Advisory Committee[44] listed several points that led them to establish field trial guidelines for the vaccine. Relevant points within the guidelines reveal the following: the amount of work involved, the testing and retesting completed, the time required, the manner in which minute details were to be accurately recorded, and the reports required to get the vaccine ready for mass testing. It was deemed unnecessary to include step-by-step technical laboratory procedures and pages of charts gauging results that would only be excitedly reviewed by immunologists, epidemiologists, and virologists. Specific requirements included:

- That research to develop a noninfectious vaccine for the prevention of paralytic poliomyelitis has been conducted by Dr. Jonas E. Salk, a grantee of the National Foundation, at the Virus Research Laboratory of the University of Pittsburgh for a period of over three years, employing more than 4,000 monkeys in testing (the) safety and antigenicity of his vaccine.

- That the Committee has held many meetings to discuss Dr. Salk's work, at six of which Dr. Salk was present and reported on the progress of his efforts and presented protocols showing the results of his work.
- That there has been developed a vaccine produced from virus of the three known types of poliomyelitis, grown in cultures of monkey kidney tissue, using Synthetic Medium 199 as a nutrient and inactivated with formalin.
- That between May 16, 1953, and March 9, 1954, Dr. Salk inoculated 5320 human beings with vaccine prepared in his own laboratory (employing most of the principles subsequently incorporated in the Specifications and Minimal Requirements), and has thereby shown the possibility of stimulating the production of poliomyelitis antibodies in the blood without causing any recognizable untoward effects upon the recipients, many of whom have had several inoculations.
- That the efficacy of the vaccine in preventing paralytic poliomyelitis in human beings under natural conditions is yet to be determined.
- That Dr. Salk is unable to undertake such an evaluation and, therefore, has requested the National Foundation, because of its resources and facilities, to assume the administrative and financial responsibility for the evaluation.
- That the National Foundation has requested the Vaccine Advisory Committee to advise it as to whether or not it should assume this administrative and financial responsibility for said evaluation.[45]

Adopted the following Resolutions:
A. That the Vaccine Advisory Committee unanimously recommends to the National Foundation that it assume the administrative and financial responsibility for evaluation of "POLIOMYELITIS VACCINE, TYPES 1, 2, AND 3."
B. That to determine the efficacy of the vaccine, in preventing paralytic poliomyelitis in human beings, the 1,401,100 cubic centimeters of vaccine already manufactured and tested pursuant to said Specifications and Minimal Requirements and any additional vaccine so manufactured and tested and approved by the Committee be used in carefully controlled evaluation studies . . . [46]

These guidelines reveal the enormous amount of preparation required to complete the field trial. There were no procedures in place for such a task, and validation was critical for acceptance by the scientific community. Newly developed specific guidelines that, allowed for the trials to be closely monitored proved extremely successful, later becoming the template for future virological studies. The field tests that adhered to these guidelines became part of the largest field trial ever held.

Salk and Sabin

During the time Salk and his team were working on his virus typing program, the egos and politics amongst the other researchers began to escalate. Salk quietly continued working simultaneously on protocols for his vaccine. Outside of Salk's laboratory, Drs. Harry Weaver and Thomas M. Rivers were the only ones aware of his clandestine efforts. Conflicts became more pronounced between Salk and Sabin. Salk was working on a method using inactivated virus[47] that contradicted Sabin's methodology. Sabin was convinced his methodology of live-virus[48] vaccine was the only accepted choice for dealing with the poliovirus. Sabin, older and already established as an excellent polio researcher, considered himself the spokesman concerning the creation of vaccines. He had also envisioned himself as the leader of those researchers who were opposed to the field trial of the Salk vaccine being planned by the NFIP. He was a strong speaker, and he talked this opposition up among his colleagues, to the Congress of the United States, in public at scientific meetings, and in letters to the NFIP. He even called Salk out publicly at a professional meeting and belittled him as a scientist. In actuality, he wanted to delay the field trials until his own vaccine was ready.

Basil O'Connor added to the bitterness and animosity between Salk, the other researchers, and the foundation by ignoring their conflicting egos.[49] Furthermore, the NFIP continued to support Sabin and others in their research. Unfortunately, Sabin continued to lead his "team" of colleagues against Salk, and Salk continued to find himself excluded from professional programs and other activities.

No amount of effort would make Salk understand why colleagues rejected his findings or insisted on delaying the tests of his work. There was no laboratory technique to discover why Parke-Davis would not follow his procedures. . . . Part of the problem was competition and jealousy. . . In the world of research scientists, a corollary to the need to publish one's findings in a scholarly journal is the insistence that new discoveries are not judged true until they have been duplicated by others. The catch was that while many people criticized Salk's work, few tried to duplicate it. Those who did seemed not to have understood what he was doing."[50] This conflict between Salk and Sabin continued for the rest of their lives.

To exacerbate things further, Weaver and others became involved in several conflicts that gave O'Connor and Salk continued frustration. Weaver wanted to direct the future field trial. In addition, he was quite rude to Dr. Hart Van Riper (1905–2000), medical director of the National Foundation.[51] This led to Weaver leaving the foundation in September 1953. O'Connor then began to direct the design of the field trial.

Salk also had a myriad of interruptions as a result of the National Foundation's announcement that a field trial was chosen, particularly the diversion of time and energy from his research because of the publicity of this research. The press wanted to interview him and his friends wanted to talk to him, making Salk feel like he was being pushed to make ready a vaccine, and he did not want to be pushed. He was just 38 years old and at the beginning of his career and was known to be enthusiastic, smart, concise, accurate, detail oriented, and honest in his reporting. He certainly could not and would not do anything that would hurt his reputation, his university, the foundation, or the children and the public he was so dedicated to helping. The vaccine was ready, but it had to undergo rigorous field trials under controlled circumstances in order to evaluate its effectiveness. Salk was not equipped to undertake such a huge project due to the needed resources. The NFIP was informed of this huge responsibility, leading them to instigate the design and implementation of the field trial and then to fund the whole project utilizing Salk's vaccine and techniques.

What Is a Field Trial?

Like any other specialized endeavor, field trials have their own vocabulary. . . . The product may be experimental, but the process of testing it is not. Trial sounds good, and a field trial is when you take the study out of the lab and into the great world—into the field. . . . A field trial is to see whether or not a new treatment or medication is safe and if it is effective . . . . Those who take part in the field trial are known as the subjects, or the test population. The investigators watch them to see if they suffer any side effects and compare their health to that of other, similar people who have not received the substance under trial. The members of this comparison group are called the controls, or the control population.
—Jane S. Smith, *Patenting the Sun*

Smith's description[52] is a simple test design. Of course, the design of the polio field trial was not simple; in fact, it was quite complex. Definitions are necessary in order to understand the process. In a blind study, the subjects receive a dose of something, whether by mouth or injection, and none of them know if they got the real substance (test dose) being tested. It could be something harmless like a sugar pill or a drink of plain water (i.e., a placebo).[53] A double-blind study is when neither the doctor nor the nurse giving the injection or dose, nor the subjects, nor anyone else involved in the field trial know who got the test dose and who got the placebo. The type of field trial design used by the NFIP was a double-blind, placebo-control study. The particular design was more complex because many more subjects must be included; the test doses and the placebos must look exactly alike; every dose of both the test dose and placebo must be coded; the codes cannot be broken into or tampered with; and records must be carefully handled and kept secret until all reports and data collection are complete. Importantly, the statistical analysis must be done by highly qualified statisticians. This insures the results are reliable and above reproach. Certainly, with so much time, money, and effort put into this project, nothing short of the most accurate results was acceptable.

Many other activities had to be completed before the field trial could take place. Test sites must be identified and approved, procedures must be clearly written, forms must be designed and printed, appropriate equipment and space must be arranged at each test site, and, finally, supplies must be ordered. Supplies for the field trial included, for example, 2.2 million sterile needles, adhesive bandages, and lollipops, which had to be divided and delivered to each test site. Very few manufacturers, in 1954, had the inventory to fulfill these needs. Finally, volunteers had to be identified and trained, public health officials in each state and community had to be contacted, and support had to be obtained; the same was true for physicians and nurses for each test site. Importantly, a method of filing and transporting the completed forms from the sites to the analysis center must be developed.

Important and critical to the success of the field trial, the parents of the children to be vaccinated were to be contacted and explanations given about the vaccine and the procedure; they must then sign a form requesting their child become a "Polio Pioneer." In order for the trial's results to be valid, a substantial number of children must have received all three of the doses. Additionally, before a decision could be made that the trial vaccine was safe and effective, two questions had to be answered: Did the child make antibodies against the three types of polioviruses included in the doses? Did the child contract polio during the later polio season that followed the field trial?[54]

Who Would Manufacture the Vaccine?

Dr. Jonas Salk became upset when he found out that Dr. Harry Weaver had made, prior to his departure from the NFIP, a verbal agreement with Parke-Davis to manufacture the vaccine. Too much was at stake. Salk felt that allowing only one manufacturer would present too many opportunities for mistakes. Therefore, O'Connor invited other manufacturers to participate. Since no vaccine was patented, it was easier for the NFIP to set conditions for the participating drug companies.[55] The NFIP's requirement for the companies who were interested was that the foundation would pay all the up-front costs of manufacturing the vaccine and then be given the vaccine at cost. At the end of the field trial, when the vaccine would be deemed safe, effective, and licensed, the manufacturer could then bring it to the public and charge its marked-up price.

Who Would Evaluate the Field Trial?

The next critical decision to be made was who would be given the responsibility for evaluating the field trial. Since there had never been a project this big, there was no previous example or procedure one could follow. One criterion for selection was that the individual could not be part of the working teams, the foundation, or the manufacturers, including no nepotism. He or she must be nonbiased in any preconceived notions, either political or technical. Basil O'Connor had to find a strong, experienced person with an impeccable research record who could direct the field trial of Salk's vaccine. He singled out Dr. Thomas Francis Jr. (1900–1969)[56] to fill that role.

Francis had been Salk's mentor. While at Francis's laboratory, Salk had begun working on flu viruses, particularly the method of preparation utilizing killed vaccines. O'Connor knew Francis had such an outstanding rating for excellence in research among his peers, and he would never be second-guessed or accused of being biased or "playing politics." So when Francis received the call from O'Connor through Dr. Hart Van Riper, he replied he had to think about all of the steps in the process and asked for more time to make his decision. Francis realized he would have to put his own research aside for the years it would take to complete the field trial report.

When Francis committed to the request, he made his own demands: he would design the field trial, have complete control of the information, and neither Salk nor O'Connor could have any influence on his report. He wanted the results to be above reproach or criticism. Furthermore, Francis demanded the study design be a double-blind field trial, with a control group of one-half of the children injected with a placebo. To be statistically valid, "a conservative approach dictated that a practical goal be set for the inoculation of between 500,000 and a million children . . . The plan adopted by the Advisory Committee of the Foundation required that each child receiving vaccine be given a series of three 1-cc injections intramuscularly at 0, 1 and 5 weeks."[57]

The field trial called for the involvement of approximately two million first through third grade school children from 217 health districts located in forty-four states.[58] This meant "there would have to be many thousands of adults helping to keep them in line."[59] The Final Report, published by the Poliomyelitis Vaccine Evaluation Center at the University of Michigan noted, "It is estimated that more than 300,000 persons, including physicians, nurses, school teachers, public health and school officials, and community volunteers recruited by National Foundation chapters and by other civic organizations cooperated in this extraordinary medical undertaking. To standardize all parts of each of the steps in the Field Trial, so that each state and community taking part would complete each step alike, a *Manual of Suggested Procedures* was prepared and used for training of participants."[60] On a specific number of children, a blood sample was drawn before the first inoculation and two weeks after the last vaccine was given in November 1954, so comparisons of antibody level (titers) could be made. The more antibodies had been made in response to the inoculations, the more effective the vaccine.[61]

Although the benefits of the vaccine would be for all people, institutional racism was evident at every level. Drs. Jonas Salk's, Albert Sabin's, and Jerome Syverton's laboratories appeared to be all white. Decisions regarding every level of the field trial were instituted and directed by white officials. Nonetheless, the NFIP would boldly break through these barriers by including black people in important roles within its organization and as part of the field trial. This plan included what Tuskegee would add in support of the study.

Who Would Receive the Vaccine: Racism and Polio

Naomi Rogers, writing in a paper published by the *Journal of American Public Health*, addressed the prevalent problem of racism within the white health community during the 1930s and 1940s that led to the belief that black people "were not susceptible to this disease, and therefore research and treatment efforts that focused on black patients were neither medically necessary nor fiscally justified."[62] She further notes: "The Tuskegee Institute opened a polio center in 1941 funded by the March of Dimes. The center's funding was the result of a new visibility of Black polio survivors and the growing political embarrassment around the policy of the Georgia Warm Springs polio rehabilitation center . . . which had maintained a Whites-only policy of admission . . . This policy, reflecting the ubiquitous norm of race-segregated health facilities, was sustained by a persuasive scientific argument about polio itself."[63] Nevertheless, black donors contributed to the fundraising activities of the March of Dimes, especially by participating in the President's Birthday Balls (figure 43) as well as the March of Dimes campaigns.[64]

Rogers further posits "during the late 1940s, in response to civil rights activism and Cold War race politics, the Foundation gradually began to use its funding to try to integrate training programs and health facilities."[65] Realistically, this was a confirmation of their own mission statement that "funds for polio treatment should be offered to all polio victims."[66] In further response to their new outreach to previously unassisted polio victims, in 1944, the NFIP hired Charles Bynum,[67] a black professional from the Office of the President at Tuskegee University, as head of the new department of Negro Activities.

Between 1944 and 1954, Bynum (figure 44) diligently worked to sway NFIP officials concerning their national health policy toward a more tolerant and inclusive policy regarding African Americans with polio.[68] He successfully in-

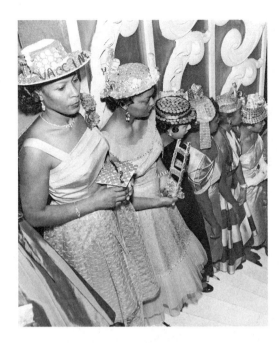

Figure 43. President's Birthday Ball at Tuskegee. (Courtesy of the Tuskegee University Archives)

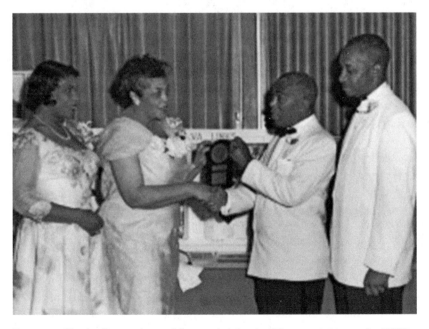

Figure 44. Charles Bynum (second from right), head of Negro activities at the NFIP. (Courtesy of the March of Dimes Archives)

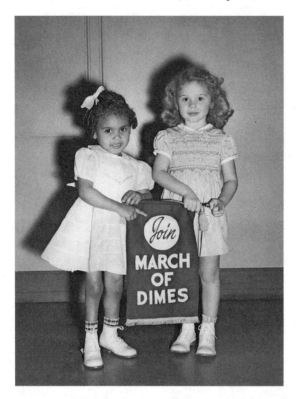

Figure 45. First NFIP poster featuring a black child, c. 1949. (Courtesy of the March of Dimes Archives)

creased "interracial fund-raising in the March of Dimes" and helped to "improve polio treatment for black Americans, and further the civil rights movement."[69] Furthermore, he utilized personal contacts to aid in advancing his agendas.

Dr. Paul B. Cornely,[70] hired as a consultant by Bynum, quickly became Bynum's confidant and collaborator. Cornely worked with him to develop a thirty-five page report to the NFIP that outlined procedures for improving polio treatment for black patients. This led to increased involvement by black communities in the NFIP, resulting in the first African American child being featured on a March of Dimes poster[71] in 1947 (figure 45); the poster was displayed primarily in black neighborhoods.[72] Empowered African Americans were soon more involved in NFIP committees.

This finally led to a national campaign poster depicting an "African American nurse caring for a white polio patient, thereby situating black medical professionals in respected positions of trust."[73] Posters such as this helped to increase awareness of African American health-care professionals as capable and caring, as well as emphasizing the fact that polio was a universal disease affecting all races, no matter their age or sex. As more people became aware "of

Black polio cases, the science of polio also shifted and the theory of polio's racial susceptibility faded."[74]

Through the efforts of Bynum and others, civil rights activists sought equality in health care with as much intensity as they had for voting rights. This led to black children being made "part of the 1954 Salk vaccine trials and the subsequent national vaccination programs."[75] There is no doubt that without the efforts of Bynum, changes in the NFIP and health care for African Americans would have been severely delayed, maybe for many years. Therefore, it is almost certain that African American children would not have been included in the polio field trials.

Bynum's ties to Tuskegee University were no accident. The longtime relationship between the Roosevelts, Basil O'Connor, and Tuskegee University led to his appointment to the NFIP. This relationship led to Tuskegee's involvement in the greatest field trial ever conducted, a field trial that would lead to a treatment for children all over the world.

The Field Trial

Most of the problems had at last been solved; the polio field trial design was finalized and an agreement had been made regarding how to proceed. All participating inoculation sites were ready and fully stocked with supplies, and volunteers had been trained. Release and "Request to Participate" forms had been signed by the parents of children who would be Polio Pioneers and were returned and placed on file at the respective sites. On April 26, 1954, the first of the series of inoculations began. One week later, the second dose was given, followed by the third dose five weeks later. The process was very precise. In fact, a field trial this extensive and exacting had never happened before and would probably never happen again. The step-by-step standard operating procedure (SOP) was utilized by health-care workers in this large field trial. These procedures were meant as a quality-control measure to protect the accuracy and validity of the project.[76]

Details were important to gauge the validity of a scientific endeavor such as this. Every contingency was anticipated in the manual. Sloppy details meant the results could be unreliable, thereby invalidating the entire field trial. The size of the field trial and the health implications for the whole world meant there were scientists from all over turning a critical eye toward its results.

Summer began after the last shots were given and the last blood samples were drawn, bringing with it polio season. It was also time to see how well the vaccine had worked. The statistical record-keeping going on inside the Polio Evaluation Center[77] was extensive. Information of all types was gathered, including cases of polio that developed after the trial had ended. Of special interest were those cases that specifically led to paralysis or death. Alton Blakeslee provides a dramatic description, noting:

Nearly 144 million separate pieces of information were collated and analyzed by Dr. Francis' team . . . Some days, the mail filled an elevator in the evaluation center's headquarters . . . everything had to [be] double-checked; a few mistakes could seriously affect the accuracy of the great conclusion. Polio cases occurring in the last months of the year of 1954 had to be included . . . From it all came the secret whether the vaccine worked. On the hope that it would prove out, pharmaceutical firms began in the 1954 to produce and stockpile vaccine, against the anticipated demand if Dr. Francis said 'Yes.' . . . he hadn't completed the analysis. He simply wasn't talking. He was ready to talk April 12, 1955. The University of Michigan and the National Foundation invited 500 prominent scientists and health leaders to hear his report . . . The Big Secret ticked loud as a time-bomb in consciousness. At 9 A.M. on Tuesday, April 12, 1955, newspapermen and photographers were waiting in a large rectangular press room . . . . on the Michigan campus. Downstairs in the auditorium, the scientific audience was filing in to hear Dr. Francis' momentous report. Not until 10:30 would he begin to read it . . . Among 440,000 vaccinated children, only 71 paralyzed by polio, but 445 paralyzed among the unvaccinated. Only 113 youngsters made sick by poliovirus, including non-paralytic cases, among the protected, but 750 among those not protected. Not a single death among those vaccinated with three shots, but 15 tragically succumbing among the non-vaccinated. No polio caused by the vaccinations, not significant reactions from the injections themselves—a safe vaccine . . . . The vaccine was about 80–90 per cent protective overall said Dr. Francis. Later in this day of Tuesday, vaccine was officially licensed for public use by the U. S. Department of Health, Education and Welfare, on recommendation of the Public Health Service after consultation with a committee of polio authorities gathered at Ann Arbor . . . . Enough vaccine was expected for 30 million children during 1955, including nine million in the first and second grades, plus some in the third grades, to be given free vaccine bought by the March of Dimes . . . The weapon had proved itself—now was the beginning of a great triumph over the ubiquitous enemy polio."[78]

Before 10:30 A.M. on April 12, 1955, the Salk vaccine belonged to the scientists in the research laboratory and the National Foundation for Infantile Paralysis;

however, by noon of the same day, the Salk vaccine belonged to the people of the United States and the world.

The trial began on April 26, 1954, involving 1.8 million children in 44 states. The cost was substantial at $25,541,662.00, or approximately $218,000,000.00 in today's money. These were voluntary contributions, meaning no taxpayer funds. Of the total, $18 million was spent on research and $7.5 million was used for the field trial. Dr. Hart Van Riper, the medical director of the March of Dimes foundation, noted in 1955, "The average American paid about 15 cents to find safe and effective means of licking polio—or less than the price of a cup of coffee and a doughnut."[79] But, there is more to this story.

Tuskegee University's role in this important study has been overlooked for far too long. Much has been written about Basil O'Connor's work in securing an Infantile Paralysis Center at Tuskegee University in 1941, where black children could get access to quality polio treatment. However, just as importantly, he facilitated the inclusion of the research scientists at the George Washington Carver Foundation in the development of the Salk vaccine. Not only was Tuskegee University's addition to the study unique in that it was one of the HBCUs, and the only institution of higher learning without a medical school, but it may have provided the only black research scientists in the project. These scientists were instrumental in supporting the mission of the NFIP by contributing cell cultures directly involved in the field trials. These cell cultures, containing HeLa cells, would definitely change the way Tuskegee's work in health-related research would continue from this point forward. This story is one of validation and vindication, that African American scientists were just as capable as their white counterparts in research and invention.

5
Tuskegee University's HeLa Cell Project

The operation at Tuskegee is very specialized indeed. There are few other organizations equipped to turn out so many HeLa cell tubes and bottles. It is interesting to note that the procedures at Tuskegee were established very rapidly to meet the need of polio research and the present evaluation of the Salk vaccine.

—Dave Preston to Charles Bynum, November 17, 1954

Tuskegee's role in the eradication of polio was significant because it was the culmination of almost fifty years of human in vitro cell experimentation. From the groundbreaking work of Hanning in 1904[1] to the efforts of Dr. John Enders in the late 1940s, work with cells had developed to the point that the NFIP felt comfortable with seeking a response to polio. Cell production, particularly HeLa cells, had reached a point where the viability of laboratory testing of Salk's and Sabin's vaccines was possible. Reaching beyond the institutional racism of the time, Tuskegee scientists produced enough HeLa cells to support 12 laboratories[2] that tirelessly worked toward testing the efficacy of the Salk vaccine. Finally, the parallel paths of the NFIP and Tuskegee University abruptly converged into one of the most important field trials ever attempted.

During this time, the use of HeLa cells was rife with moral dilemmas such as those so extensively revealed by Rebecca Skloot's book, *The Immortal Life of Henrietta Lacks*.[3] The cells were obtained by Dr. George Otto Gey[4] from a terminally ill cancer patient named Henrietta Lacks. Lacks suffered from cervical cancer,[5] from which she died in 1951. These cells were the first successful in vitro human cell line and eventually proved to be profoundly beneficial to medical research; all of this without the knowledge, until recently, of anyone within her family. At that time, informed consent was not required to use her cells.

However, concern for a patient's rights is not a modern concept. In 1905, the US Supreme Court cited that citizen's rights prohibited "a physician or surgeon, however skilled or eminent . . . to violate without permission the bodily integrity of his patient . . . and [to operate] on him without his consent or knowledge."[6] In 1914, the court made it an assault if a physician failed to notify a patient of intent to operate. By the late 1950s, patients had acquired the right to know of the potential positive or negative effects of a physician's actions. Although these rulings were broadened to include a variety of specific cases, it was not until 1972 that physicians were required to disclose medical risks in language patients could understand.[7] The California Supreme Court's decision in *Cobbs v. Grant* (1972) declared, the "scope of the disclosure required of physicians defies simple definition" and must "be measured by the patient's need, and that need is whatever information is material to the decision."[8] Specifically, the physician must, in layman's language, provide any and all information pertinent to the patient's comprehension of their diagnosis and treatment.

Jessica De Bord, writing in an article titled "Informed Consent" for the website *Ethics in Medicine* (University of Washington School of Medicine) defines informed consent as "the process by which the treating health care provider discloses appropriate information to a competent patient so that the patient may make a voluntary choice to accept or refuse treatment. It originates from the legal and ethical right the patient has to direct what happens to her body and from the ethical duty of the physician to involve the patient in her health care."[9] The problem is that this current philosophy developed many years after the events surrounding Henrietta Lacks and her amazing cells. In spite of this apparent progress, these actions did not address the loophole of what happens to the "leftovers;" namely, the tissues, blood samples, etc., arising from day-to-day hospital operations. Current information indicates "a conservative estimate . . . that more than 307 million tissue specimens from more than 178 million cases are stored in the United States."[10]

The techniques developed during the search for the polio vaccine, including the work with the HeLa cells, led to the explosion of cell culture exploitation. However, during the time of Lacks and the polio vaccine, the issue of patient consent for the use of their cells or tissues in research was nonexistent. As Skloot concluded, "When I tell people the story of Henrietta Lacks and her cells, their first question is usually, 'Wasn't it illegal for doctors to take Henrietta's cells without her knowledge? Don't doctors have to tell you when they use your cells in research?' The answer is no—not in 1951, and not in 2009, when this book went to press."[11]

During a biopsy, Dr. Howard Jones at Johns Hopkins Hospital in Baltimore, Maryland, recognized Lacks's cancer as particularly unique, describing it as "shining and purple like grape jello."[12] The biopsied sample was sent to the pathology lab for diagnosis. The result confirmed stage one cancer of the cervix. Jones's boss, Dr. Richard Wesley TeLinde, one of the top cervical cancer specialists in the country, attempted to prove his theory that both carcinoma in situ and invasive carcinoma were basically the same form of cancer and should be treated the same by seeking cells specifically from indigent cancer patients with cervical cancer, including Lacks. TeLinde worked with Gey to grow the cancer cells in his lab, seeking to collaborate with each other to examine the cells in order to determine their similarities. Gey had other research goals; he and his wife, Dr. Margaret K. Gey, were determined to find and grow the first "immortal" human cells for research.

After Lacks was anesthetized as part of her first radium treatment on February 8, 1951, Dr. Lawrence Wharton Jr., removed "two dime sized pieces of tissue from her cervix; one from her tumor and one from healthy tissue nearby."[13] The samples were then taken to the Geys' laboratory. Amazingly, over the next few days, the cancerous cells began to replicate at a phenomenal rate. The Geys had done it; they had found the first immortal cells. After appearing on a local television program, Gey announced to the world his results, three weeks after Lacks began her radiation treatment. Later, he began shipping the cells all over the country, including to the laboratories of Drs. Jerome T. Syverton, William F. Scherer, and Jonas Salk. On October 4, 1951, Lacks passed away due to complications with cancer, but her cells continued to live on as the now-famous HeLa cells. It is important to note the use of her cells played a major role in the triumph of the Salk vaccine. Tuskegee's involvement would prove to be instrumental in the immortality of those cells.

The reasons for choosing Tuskegee over other laboratories associated with large medical research-focused institutions such as Duke, Vanderbilt, Johns Hopkins, or MD Anderson are partially due to the well-known history of both Booker T. Washington and the legacy of the George Washington Carver Research Foundation (GWCRF).[14] In addition, Basil O'Connor had an intimate knowledge of the research being conducted at the GWCRF and noted during a speech given in November 1950: "we must continue to broaden the field of opportunity to make places for our best brains, our most capable hands, our most dynamic personalities, whether they be Negro or white," for "as a nation, we cannot continue to squander the abilities of our people without lessening our capacity for world leadership."[15] The confidence both Bynum and O'Connor had in the capability of Tuskegee's scientists confirms this.

The Work Begins

The year 1952 was a momentous one: the new George Washington Carver Research building at Tuskegee was completed; Dr. George Otto Gey and his co-workers had isolated the cell strain known as HeLa; and Dr. Jonas Salk had completed the virus typing program. Salk confirmed there were only three types of poliovirus that would need to be included in the vaccine. He had also completed the design and preliminary testing of the vaccine and was now ready to test its efficacy. The plans and design of the field trial by the NFIP were already in progress.

It was recognized from the start that an orderly laboratory program was essential if the objectives of the investigations were to be achieved. "At a meeting of investigators held in Chicago in March of 1954, plans for the Field Trial and earlier recommendations were presented, laboratory techniques were discussed in detail, and agreement was reached upon standard procedures to be employed."[16] Data presented in February 1954 had already "indicated that monkey kidney epithelial cells and HeLa cell type cultures were equally good for the detection of virus in stool specimens. Dr. Julius S. Younger, a partner in Salk's laboratory, developed a colorimetric test to be used as an indicator in titrating poliomyelitis virus or its antibody, using the monkey kidney cell system. Dr. Jerome Syverton also discussed the usefulness of HeLa cells as indicators of poliomyelitis virus or its antibody . . . It was agreed, however, that either HeLa or monkey kidney epithelial cells could be used in suspended or stationary cultures for titration of antibody; a schedule of dilutions of serum and concentration of virus was adopted."[17]

Everything was in place for the work to begin. The time span for the trials was 1952 to 1955. It must be remembered that a concerted effort involving research by a large number of biomedical scientists culminated in the development of two effective polio vaccines. The first was the Salk vaccine containing inactivated virus, and the second was the Sabin vaccine containing attenuated virus. The technology that made these vaccines possible was a composite of a number of significant contributions. Tuskegee's efforts in this endeavor revolved around the Salk vaccine. In fact, Tuskegee's "project established that it is feasible to mass produce cultures" of cells making "it the forerunner of the current commercial production in the United States and in other countries."[18]

During preliminary consultations, it appeared the needed supply of primate cells had become questionable and a host-cell alternative was necessary. The primate cells often originated in underdeveloped countries and needed to be placed in a location that would act as a clearinghouse, ensuring they were free from any viruses. This required an extended stay in a reliable facility. In a memorandum to Dr. Van Riper at the NFIP from Dr. Weaver, he states:

> I have just returned from a conference on tissue culture with our grantees. The conference recommended that we take steps to have produced a continuing supply of standard tissue culture tubes which can be shipped to the various laboratories as needed. One of these tubes will, for many experiments, be equivalent to one monkey. It is estimated that as many as 20,000 such tubes per week might be needed. The service proposed is essentially similar to that now being rendered the grantees through Okatie Farms[19] except that in this case it relates not to monkeys, but to standard tissue culture tubes. Present plans are to make such tubes from

monkey testes. The magnitude of this job is apparent from the facts that one technician can make approximately 500 such tubes per day and that one pair of monkey testes will provide sufficient tests to make approximately 300 such tubes.

There were two important problems at that time with using monkeys for development of the vaccine. First, there was an insufficient supply of monkey cells due to other processes recently developed, such as the Rh blood factor research. As the letter from Dr. Weaver stated, there were not enough primate cells to meet the demands of the field trial. Limited numbers of viable primates would hinder the test, as well as the development of the vaccine. Fewer primates meant higher costs. This alone could have stopped the test. Second, as Dr. Van Riper noted in a letter to O'Connor, dated May 27, 1952, due to "the changing picture of research" there was "a lessening need for monkeys in any large numbers. Because of these factors, Basil O'Connor made a handwritten note on a memorandum from Weaver: "Tuskegee to take over whole operation. BOC 10.6.52."[20] Strain HeLa was selected as an alternative to the primates, and the NFIP decided it would be expedient to establish Tuskegee University as a central source of supply.

Russell Brown and Jimmy Henderson

Regarding the choice of Tuskegee University as a "central source," two Tuskegee University research scientists, Drs. Russell Brown and James (Jimmy) Henderson, writing in a then-unpublished paper titled *The Ubiquitous HeLa Cell: Historic Account of the Mass Production and Distribution of HeLa Cells at Tuskegee Institute, 1953–1955*,[21] stated:

It is of historical interest to relate how Tuskegee Institute, which had no previous involvement or expertise in animal cell culture, was selected to undertake the HeLa project. It was the desire of NFIP that this particular project conform to the protocol developed by the National foundation, as articulated by Dr. H. M. Weaver, Director of Research, and that this could be accommodated best by a university having personnel and an organization with experience in accepting a flexible range of research and development projects. Dr. Weaver was personally acquainted with Tuskegee Institute and especially the activities of the Carver Research Foundation (CRF), and he discussed the need for a central HeLa production laboratory with Dr. Russell Brown, CRF Director, in October 1952 and it was agreed, subsequently, that the project would be awarded to Tuskegee Institute . . . It was decided that Brown would serve as principal investigator (PI) with the assistance of James H. M. Henderson. It was arranged by Weaver for Brown and Henderson to spend three months and six weeks, respectively, studying cell and tissue culture methods under the supervision of William F. Scherer and Jerome T. Syverton, Department of Microbiology, School of Medicine, University of Minnesota, Minneapolis, January 1953 through March 1953. Following this period of study, Scherer was engaged by NFIP as consultant for the project and J. Newton Ashworth, Director of the Blood Program, American Red Cross, served as advisor on packaging and shipping.

Although there are inconsistencies within their account,[22] Brown and Henderson provide another piece to the puzzle regarding the selection of Tuskegee. The emphasis on Weaver's knowledge of Tuskegee is based upon Brown and Henderson's relationship to the scientific community. In fact, that relationship shows the respect, during a time of segregation and institutional racism, given to Tuskegee's research scientists by others throughout the nation.

Ironically, it was to Tuskegee the NFIP turned in the 1940s and again in the 1950s as an important center for scientific and cultural knowledge and as a service to the African American community. Why not turn to a white institution, previously experienced in laboratory research? And if not a white institution, why not Meharry Medical College or the prestigious Hampton University? What made Tuskegee a desirable location for such an important project? Primarily, it was the intimate relationship between the NFIP and Tuskegee that led to the important decision to construct and utilize a modern and up-to-date research facility for the propagation and mass distribution of the HeLa cells.

Early in the 1940s, the NFIP established on the Tuskegee University Campus the Infantile Paralysis Center as a critically needed treatment center for African American children with polio, the only such facility in the nation. It is during the Salk vaccine field trials in the early 1950s the NFIP would again turn to Tuskegee for the replication of the HeLa cells. The NFIP provided a niche for Tuskegee as a significant contributor to meeting not only their mandate but also the mandates of Booker T. Washington and George W. Carver.

The project at Tuskegee was to be overseen by Brown,[23] initially assisted by Henderson.[24] Brown (figure 46) was the director of the Carver Research Foundation (CRF), and Henderson was a researcher working with cell cultures involving sunflower tumors and related plant tissues. Brown had shown a propensity for venturing into new directions as a scientist and researcher. He worked in a variety of positions during his tenure at Tuskegee (1936–1970), serving as a researcher in microbiology and biochemistry, as well as a variety

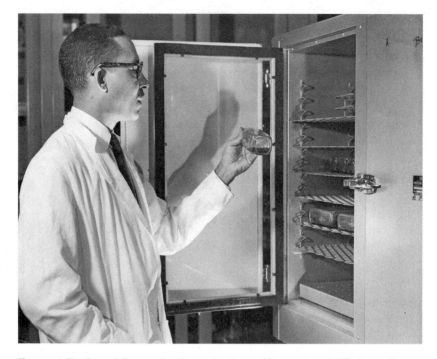

Figure 46. Dr. Russell Brown checking cell cultures. (Courtesy of the Tuskegee University Archives)

of academic and administrative positions. Henderson was persuaded to join Brown because of his knowledge and research experience with plant tissue cell culture.

It was Brown who approached Dr. Frederick D. Patterson, then Tuskegee's president, regarding support for the project. In a letter to Weaver, dated November 21, 1952, Brown indicated: "I have discussed with President Patterson the proposal concerning the preparation of tissue culture and media. I am happy to advise that he is strongly in favor of us undertaking the program and he has granted approval for us to go ahead with it."[25] Later, on February 10, 1953, Brown spoke before the Annual Meeting of the Board of Directors of the George Washington Carver Foundation announcing "we are beginning a new project with the National Foundation for Infantile Paralysis . . . in a venture that will not lose money."[26] This was important for Tuskegee; not only would they receive prestige and honor for the work to be performed, they would do the work without any financial liability. In fact, Dr. Roy C. Newton,[27] CRF Board member, commented that, "the selection of the Carver Foundation was highly complementary and that this venture [would] offer an opportunity to come into immediate contact with the large research organizations, thereby adding to its prestige,"[28] perhaps, adding to their financial coffers as well.

The NFIP selected Drs. Jerome Syverton and William Scherer at the University of Minnesota School of Medicine for the training of Brown and Henderson in the techniques of HeLa cell culture. Again, it was Syverton and Scherer, along with Gey, who were largely responsible for working with strain HeLa in the vaccine evaluation process. Moreover, Scherer was well known for his expertise in animal cell culture—not only through his research but also through his service on the staff of the Tissue Culture course taught at the Mary Imogene Bassett Hospital, Cooperstown, New York, from 1949 to 1953.[29]

Although Brown and Henderson were originally supposed to spend "three months and six weeks, respectively" for training at the Syverton-Scherer research complex at the University of Minnesota, Brown actually spent four weeks and Henderson two.[30] Brown returned for further training at a later date.

In a letter to Weaver regarding the training received by the two Tuskegee researchers, Scherer and Syverton noted: "The utilization of cellular cultures for virus work was demonstrated, though not actually carried out by either Drs. Russell Brown or Jimmy Henderson. Dr. Henderson participated in the preliminary exercises and observed the methods for cultivation of cells in suspension (including strain HeLa) but stayed insufficient time to perform these technics [sic]. During the last two weeks of Dr. Brown's stay, he concentrated his efforts on methods for cultivating strain HeLa. He became fully familiar with all the technics used in this and in Dr. Gey's laboratories."[31] It is possible Henderson felt his work in plant cell cultures was sufficient for this project, but it is obvious Scherer and Syverton felt otherwise. Henderson is no longer mentioned in any further project correspondence, although he later helped write about Tuskegee's work with strain HeLa.[32]

Small Training Laboratory

Scherer and Syverton emphasized the urgency of the project and Tuskegee's involvement. Brown was made aware of the "type of physical facility required, including laboratory furniture, various items of large and small equipment, especially air-conditioning, air-filtration, and relative isolation of the space used for production and handling of cell cultures."[33] Upon Brown's return to Tuskegee, a space for the cell production laboratory was sought, with Brown's research laboratory in the newly constructed Carver Research Foundation building initially chosen as a training laboratory. The location of the larger cell production laboratory was coordinated at Tuskegee with the help of Dr. Clarence T. Mason, later interim director of the CRF.[34]

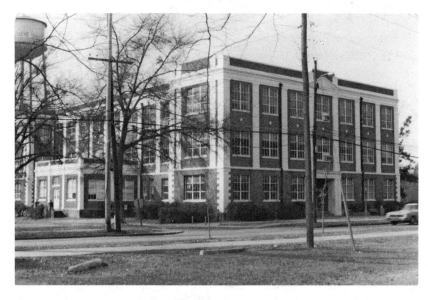

Figure 47. Armstrong Hall Laboratory located off of Old Montgomery Road. (Courtesy of the Tuskegee University Archives)

Settling on Armstrong Hall (figure 47) as the location of the new production laboratory, "renovations indicated were made, all of the basic equipment was procured and installed, and recruitment of personnel was initiated."[35] Located on the ground floor and adjacent to the CRF building, the laboratory area was large and spacious. Of importance, Armstrong Hall was the biology/chemistry building, providing an environment conducive to research and development.

The first employee hired in this new venture was Norma Gaillard (figure 48), a graduate of North Carolina Central University. She came to Tuskegee in pursuit of her master's degree in organic chemistry, graduating in 1948. Gaillard was instructed in basic cell and tissue culture techniques.

Following Gaillard, and with her assistance, four additional science graduates, Evelyn Carmon, Gloria Maxwell, George C. Busby, and Angela G. DuBose, were hired and trained as cell culture technicians. In addition, undergraduate students from well-known schools, who were also residents of Tuskegee and home for summer vacation, were likewise trained and employed, including Joan Brown, Ann Dibble, and Robert Dibble.[36] Joan Brown was Dr. Russell Brown's niece, while Ann and Robert Dibble were children of Dr. Eugene Dibble, then medical director of the John A. Andrew Memorial Hospital.

Working in the small laboratory located at the CRF, Gaillard continued with the HeLa cell culture procedures instituted by Scherer and Syverton

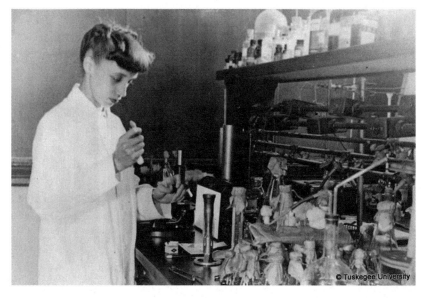

Figure 48. Norma Gaillard, cell and tissue culture technician. (Courtesy of the Tuskegee University Archives)

via Dr. Russell Brown. Other procedures Brown and Gaillard tested and improved included feeding, maintaining (figure 49), and transporting the cultures to grantee laboratories.

Because of the uniqueness of this endeavor and the fact that it had never been attempted on such a scale, it was critical for procedures to be standardized for consistency and reliability. Feeding of the cultures included factors such as proper solution formulas (or recipes), amounts required, types of containers needed, and the regularity of feeding (figure 50). Due to the location of the laboratory in south central Alabama, heat and humidity were always a major concern. Also, contamination was an ever-present issue. However, it was transportation from Tuskegee to the grantee laboratories that required the most diligent deliberation. Grantee laboratories were scattered throughout the nation, and the cultures required constant temperature control to assure they were viable upon arrival at their final destination.

Concurrently, in April 1953, Scherer brought to Tuskegee a culture of strain HeLa, which was subsequently expanded and stored as stock cultures in bottles kept in the smaller training laboratory. It was from such bottles that test tube cultures were prepared for experimental shipping (figure 51). During this visit and the many others that followed, HeLa project consultant Scherer made additional suggestions regarding specialized equipment needs and assisted in the training of Gaillard.

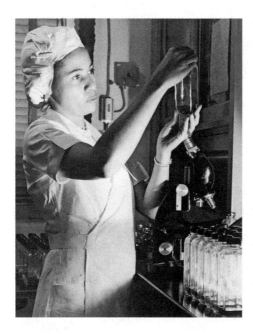

Figure 49. Jeanne M. Walton examining HeLa cells. (Courtesy of the Tuskegee University Archives)

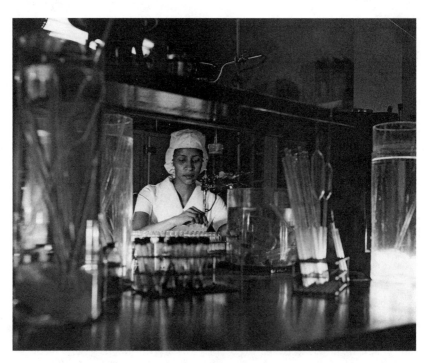

Figure 50. Technician in the Cell Culture Laboratory. (Courtesy of the Tuskegee University Archives)

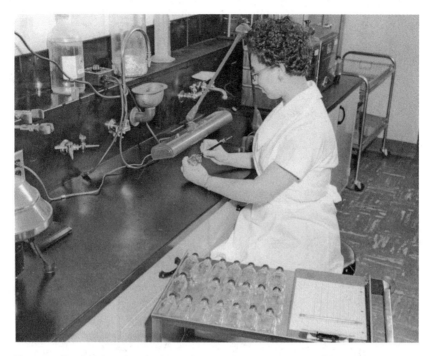

Figure 51. Stock culture bottles being examined by lab technician. (Courtesy of the Tuskegee University Archives)

Beginning on May 8, 1953, an initial experimental shipment of cultures was made to Scherer's and Salk's laboratories.[37] Not only did Scherer visit Tuskegee on a regular basis, but Weaver also visited occasionally, writing during the first week in May that he was pleased with the laboratory's progress. Furthermore, he offered helpful suggestions for moving ahead on an accelerated schedule. Weaver proposed a detailed schedule beginning May 11, 1953, which included: (1) experimental shipments of cells to Scherer; (2) occasional shipments to Dr. Jonas Salk, University of Pittsburgh; Dr. Joseph Smadel, Army Medical School; and Dr. Joseph Melnick, Yale University; and (3) the suggestion that every effort be made to develop the capacity to permit the shipment of at least 10,000 cultures per week, beginning June 1, 1953, to an expanded list of laboratories to be coordinated by Scherer.[38]

The Main Production Laboratory

In the spring of 1953, renovation of the main production laboratory located in Armstrong Hall was nearing completion. Immediately, problems dealing with the procurement of supplies began to arise. The need for large quantities of

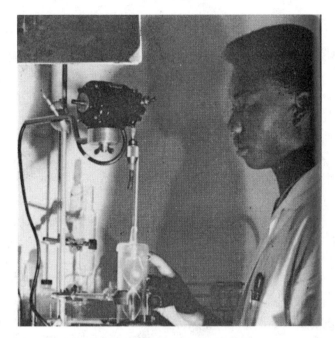

Figure 52. Joseph Jackson helping to produce HeLa cells.
(Courtesy of the Tuskegee University Archives)

items, such as test tubes, highlighted Tuskegee's and the NFIP's concerns. By July 31, 1953, logistical problems were alleviated and the production facility became fully operational. The rapid procurement of laboratory supplies was due to direct negotiations, resulting from the uninterrupted monetary involvement of the NFIP. Large quantities of expendable and special delivery items[39] led to the employment of an "expediter" specializing in the procurement of supplies.[40]

The HeLa production laboratory accommodated ten cell culture technicians and a laboratory supervisor (figure 52). Formal training resulted in personnel (figure 53) thoroughly indoctrinated in cell culture procedures specific to strain HeLa and the shipping of the cultures to grantees. They were further trained in security measures essential to the avoidance of contamination and other operational difficulties. Likewise, auxiliary personnel were given similar instructions with particular emphasis on precautions necessary to insure successful operation of the total project.[41]

The facility consisted of two sections and was designed to be air-conditioned, including an efficient air filtration system. Air purity was monitored by observing the microbial colony counts on agar plates on each bench of the cell culture section (figure 54).[42] Brown and Henderson describe the facility as follows: "Separate space and equipment provisions were made for auxiliary operations such as: cleaning and sterilization of glassware and utensils; packag-

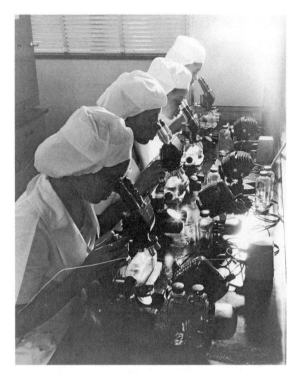

Figure 53. Technicians working in main laboratory.
(Courtesy of the Tuskegee University Archives)

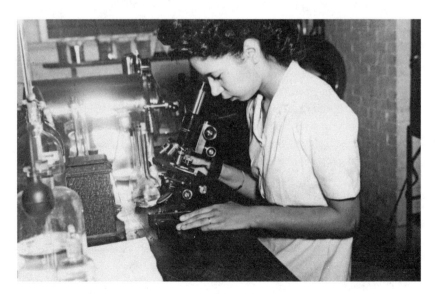

Figure 54. Technician performing colony count. (Courtesy of the Tuskegee University
Archives)

ing of the finished products (tube and bottle cultures); and for orderly storage of data resulting from day-to-day operation. The tissue culture section contained a microscope bench with several binocular microscopes which would accommodate microscopic examination of monolayer cultures in both tubes and bottles, with the use of low and high power objectives; inverted microscopes were not yet available. Microscopic examination was a routine quality control of cell morphology and of the monolayers prior to packaging for shipment."[43]

After construction, the facility was not without problems. Besides issues with acquiring supplies and training staff, there were concerns with the installed air conditioning and equipment placement.

However, problems with the facility were not the only potential impediments to the operation. During the early stages, Dr. Russell Brown was director of the Carver Research Foundation (CRF) and the principle investigator (PI) for the Salk vaccine field trial cell production project. This was very problematic. In a letter from Dr. Henry W. Kumm,[44] the new director of research at the NFIP, Scherer wrote, "As you can see, I think it is obvious that we must stop trying to make ourselves believe that Dr. Brown can or will direct this project *at the production and laboratory level.* A new professional director is needed who can and will spend full time on the project."[45] Brown's responsibilities at Tuskegee University were numerous and time consuming, leaving little time to be particularly devoted to any single project. The timelines set by the NFIP, however, required intense dedication, and the needs for such an endeavor did not make it easy for someone as overextended as Brown. This project was too big, both prestigiously and monetarily, for Brown or Tuskegee University to take lightly.

This terse letter prompted Brown to respond in December 1953, "I have assumed full time responsibility for directing the project here at Tuskegee." At this time Dr. Clarence T. Mason took on the position of interim director of the CRF. Even though Brown assumed the role of PI on a full-time basis, he nonetheless planned to resume his previous duties as soon as "the project [was] clearly under control and has been operating smoothly for a reasonable period of time." The uncertainty on the part of Brown and the Tuskegee administration no doubt caused some concern with the leadership of the NFIP.

Doubt, especially at this critical juncture of the project, was unacceptable. Scherer sought other locations in case Tuskegee proved unreliable. In a letter addressed to Kumm, Scherer noted "on my way to Alabama, I stopped to visit Microbiological Associates[46] on Sunday, January 17, 1954." This laboratory proved to be unacceptable, mainly because they would not permit "careful control of . . . production methods" by the NFIP scientists.[47] Quality control of the laboratory's procedures was of the utmost importance. In early February 1954, Kumm wrote to Scherer about his relief "to know that you now feel that the project in Alabama is in better condition than previously."[48] The corre-

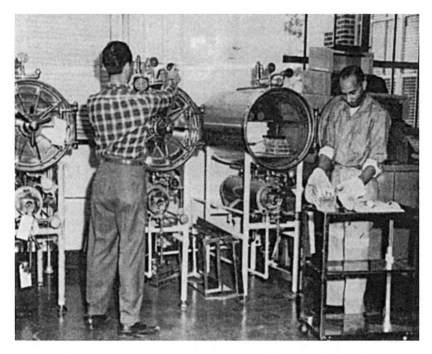

Figure 55. Autoclave in use. (Courtesy of the Tuskegee University Archives)

spondence between Scherer and his superiors reveals his deliberate intention to keep Tuskegee viable during the field trials.

However, in mid-February of the same year, Scherer was notified by a discouraged Brown of "the very serious contamination now present in the production lab." Through human error, after repeated discussions,[49] contamination had entered the laboratory through using "unsterile glassware (i.e., undoubtedly never autoclaved[50])."[51] Although it was just one batch of HeLa culture involved, it caused a sizable delay in beginning shipments of cell cultures to the grantees. After resolving the issues of contamination brought about by a variety of problems, which was attributed primarily to a breach of protocol within the laboratory, they were ready to start meeting their objective. Subsequently reviewing and implementing autoclaving procedures (figure 55), Brown later wrote, "we will very shortly be able to make enough tubes to complete the shipping experiments which Dr. Scherer and I were conducting."

This is confirmed by Dr. Syverton, in a letter written in March 1954 to Dr. Francis, who stated, "Tuskegee undoubtly [sic] can provide cells on glass in bottles to laboratories within a wide range of supply."[52] Success was attained at Tuskegee through the perseverance of NFIP officials and the professionalism of the Tuskegee staff. The NFIP and its partners had chosen well.

By late February, the laboratory had achieved the projected level of production, and it was then possible to supply the needs of the 23 field trial laboratories.[53] From April through September 1954, "approximately 133,000 tube cultures and 1,800 bottle cultures of HeLa were sent out."[54] This quantity of material was enormous and on an unprecedented scale, and a project of this nature had never been attempted. During this time, scientists at Tuskegee University, working with the Salk vaccine field trials, overcame many problems with unique solutions.

Specialized equipment was needed in response to the unique situation of mass production of the cultures. Some of the equipment required adaptations as simple as changing from test tube and bottle screw caps with pasteboard liners to rubber liners, making them airtight. This facilitated a reduction in leakage and the unlikely possibility of contamination from outside sources. The tubes were held in a specially designed rack designed by Scherer "in collaboration with the metal working firm Seeley Craftsmen of Minneapolis."[55] Made of stainless steel, the tubes were held in place from washing to inoculation and incubation through medium removal and recharging without multiple handlings. Scherer would continue to use these racks until his death in May 1982.

Other solutions were not as simple, such as the automatic dispenser assembly (figure 56) for adding nutrient-rich medium to the culture tubes. Initially, the laboratory worked with a Cornwall[56] finger-controlled "device which could be adjusted to deliver a measured volume of cell suspension."[57] In order to facilitate more accurate dispensing in a timely manner to the larger quantity HeLa culture tubes, Scherer and the laboratory scientists at Tuskegee devised a device "for delivering small volumes of cell suspension to large numbers of tubes under relatively aseptic conditions."[58] Therefore, the new assembly also helped alleviate problems specific to contamination within the laboratory.

The biggest problem during the project consisted of shipping the cultures to the respective testing laboratories. Laboratories were located throughout the nation with the furthest situated some 2,200 miles away at the University of California Medical Center in Los Angeles, California. This posed a serious problem for the Tuskegee laboratory. Not only was the distance pronounced, but in 1954 they were shipping from April through September, the hottest time of the year in the South. The cultures required a temperature range from 36 to 40 degrees centigrade throughout the entire time they were en route. Initially, the Tuskegee scientists looked to ship the HeLa cultures via buses, which proved unreliable due to inconsistent arrivals and departures. Airplanes proved to be the most reliable mode of transportation, but after much trial and error, it was determined the cultures needed special handling.[59] Boxes were labeled "PERISHABLE BIOLOGICAL MATERIAL," and the carriers were instructed to avoid excessive heat or cold. The packages containing the HeLa cultures were taken "directly to the Columbus, Georgia or to the Montgomery, Alabama airports in time for prearranged regular air express flights with the

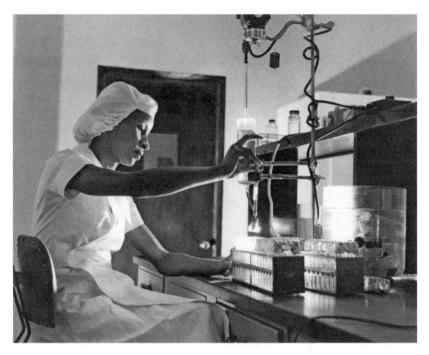

Figure 56. Technician Joyce Perry utilizing assembly in dispensing HeLa cells. (Courtesy of the Tuskegee University Archives)

most favorable long distance connections."[60] The objective was to keep the time frame for delivery limited to a maximum of two days.[61] Furthermore, in a letter from Dr. Hart Van Riper to Basil O'Connor, dated October 22, 1953, it was noted: "Post office conditions at Tuskegee Institute are not satisfactory and it has been recommended that the Institute deliver the tubes directly into Montgomery."[62] After stringent evaluations, shipping techniques were adjusted in order to provide more efficient delivery times.

To further complicate matters, the shipping containers had to be specially designed in order to ensure safe transport. The containers needed to be resilient and the proper size to accommodate the racks of culture tubes. They initially sought a shipping container that was non-returnable, possibly containing 450 culture tubes, and using phosphate salts to absorb heat, keeping the cultures within optimum temperature.

On the recommendation of Drs. Maria Telkes,[63] of New York University, and J. N. Ashworth,[64] assistant Director of the Blood Program of the American Red Cross, the Tuskegee scientists settled on a design for the most acceptable container (figure 57).[65] The final design was similar to the container used by the American Red Cross to ship blood throughout the nation. The box, measuring sixteen inches on all sides, was designed with two inches of fiberglass insula-

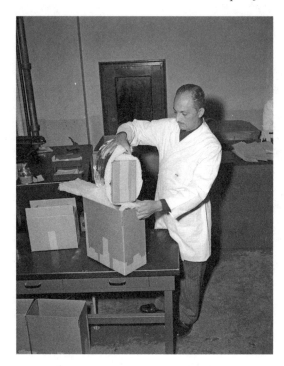

Figure 57. HeLa Cells in
a box with an equitherm
warmer. (Courtesy of the
March of Dimes Archives)

tion and able to hold 450 tubes. Optimum temperature was maintained using fusion salts in a 12 × 12 × 2 in. sealed tin can. The types of fusion salts differed between winter and summer.[66]

After the Tuskegee laboratory met all the standards instituted by the NFIP for the trials, various laboratories were selected to test the shipping cartons and techniques. In October 1954, they started sending shipments to the testing laboratories (figure 58), accompanied with a standard questionnaire to determine quality of the HeLa cultures upon receipt.

Designed by the GWCF, the questions were:

1. With cultures of optimum quality in either case, which would you consider preferable, monkey kidney or HeLa cells? Briefly state the reasons for your preference.
2. Have you received and tried HeLa cell cultures from Tuskegee since April 1 of this year? If so, were they tube cultures, bottle cultures or both?
3. If you have received shipments from Tuskegee, were the cultures all in good condition on arrival? If not, what was the difficulty (contamination, cultures past the optimum stage for use, or other)? Please indicate how frequently such deficiencies occurred.[67]

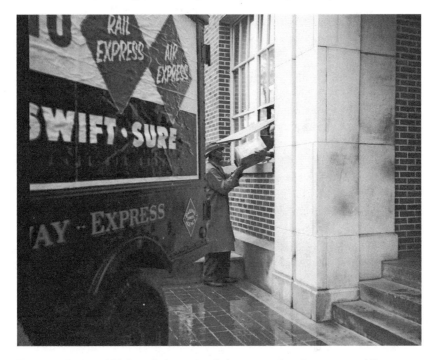

Figure 58. Packaged HeLa cells being handed out a window for transport. (Courtesy of the March of Dimes Archives)

This proved helpful to the scientists. Many of the laboratories responded that their samples proved to be contaminated due to a variety of factors. Early problems of contamination are frequent during a new procedure. Issues received quick response and resolution.

Furthermore, some of the laboratories were already using the monkey kidney cells and did not wish to change to the use of HeLa cultures. This would require instituting new procedures, retraining of technicians, and purchasing new equipment. Others received the HeLa cultures and were happy to use them. Responses to the questionnaire aided the Tuskegee scientists to determine how much material they would be required to prepare and ship on a consistent basis during the trial evaluation. The questionnaire would continue to morph into a more exhaustive format in order to facilitate better and accurate service.[68] Quality control at the Tuskegee laboratory was substantially enhanced by the knowledge received through the questionnaires.

Dr. Russell Brown was able to determine, from one of the questionnaires, that some of the HeLa cultures that arrived at the grantee laboratories in a contaminated state were in fact the result of not following the proper protocol.

First of all, some of the laboratories in question had not tested for contamination, though they reported it as such. Others were contaminated as a result of not applying the needed nutrients in a timely manner. Cultures were shipped with a separate solution of nutrient-rich medium to be added upon arrival prior to incubation and use. Failure to follow this procedure led to a variety of problems. If the medium was not added in a timely manner, the cells would be reduced in number. Furthermore, the nutrient-rich medium could have appeared cloudy, leading the grantee laboratories to assume contamination.

In a particular instance, Brown wrote to T. E. Boyd that the laboratory of Dr. Gordon C. Brown reported "that the cells in many of the tubes . . . had become dislodged from the glass surface and that he suspected contamination."[69] He immediately called the laboratory and spoke with Assistant Director Dr. D. E. Craig who reported "that some of the tubes were cloudy and were considered to be contaminated . . . but that no contaminants were actually demonstrated." Craig also reported the HeLa cultures were not immediately given the nutrient-rich medium, but were put in the incubator on arrival without being opened until the next day." This resulted in the cells not being exposed to the nutrient medium for three to four days since leaving the Tuskegee laboratory. Brown goes on to say: "it is highly probable; therefore, that the condition described . . . is attributable to the age of the culture and the manner of handling rather than to the possibility of contamination."[70] This type of follow-up was typical of Brown's dedication to the quality and success of the project.

Brown, in the conclusion to his draft "The Ubiquitous HeLa Cell: Historic Account of the Mass Production and Distribution of HeLa Cells at Tuskegee Institute, 1953–1955," matter-of-factly writes: "many laboratories were glad to obtain HeLa cultures and the number requesting HeLa eventually increased. By 30 June 1955, we had shipped approximately 600,000 cultures."[71] This was an amazing number, accomplished by a small southern laboratory located in the segregated Deep South.

All of this was done in a very short time, in a rush to find a preventive for one of the most debilitating and feared diseases of the twentieth century. Brown realized the impact of the work, but he had not considered how the work impacted black-white relations within the scientific community. He noted, in the last paragraph, "In retrospect, it was largely fortuitous that we at Tuskegee Institute had the opportunity to become involved in a program that has had such momentous growth in more recent decades."[72] It was more than fortune or luck, it was the result of a concerted effort by many people, black and white, working together for a common good, reaching beyond the ugliness of racism and segregation, and achieving something more than physical healing.

6
After the Polio Vaccine

A sound social philosophy of every race is the cultivation of the good
will of those among whom they live, rather than cherishing the hope that
somebody a thousand miles away will come and affect their deliverance.

—Booker T. Washington

The polio vaccine trials ushered in a new era in cell culture manipulation. Two
years prior to the vaccine's availability, polio affected over 45,000 people annually in the United States. Within seven years, the yearly number in the United
States had dropped to 910. The worldwide numbers of reported cases of the
virus dropped even more significantly. Currently, polio remains endemic in
three countries: Afghanistan, Nigeria, and Pakistan.[1] Millions have benefited
throughout the world from the Salk and Sabin polio vaccines. In 1956, approximately 8,000 first and second Salk vaccine injections were given to children of
Macon County (figure 59).[2] The work of thousands of anonymous people went
into the development of a disease prevention, and these stories of their commitment and sacrifices are rarely repeated.[3]

One such commonly overlooked individual is Dr. Hilary Koprowski.[4] While
working at Lederle Labs in Bound Brook, New Jersey, he created what is ar-
guably the world's first polio vaccine. Working with attenuated (rendered non-
virulent) live viruses, Koprowski was convinced live viruses could provide lifelong
immunity without the need for booster shots. The vaccine was administered
orally and was initially tested between January 1948 and February 1950. The
first patient was Koprowski himself who suffered no ill effects. Later in 1950, he
tested his vaccine on 20 children at Letchworth Village, then a home for mentally disabled children in Rockland County, New York; of those orally given the
vaccine, seventeen developed antibodies to the poliovirus without complications. Koprowski determined three of the children had already developed antibodies, thus not needing the vaccine. His vaccine was later administered to approximately two hundred and fifty thousand individuals in the Belgian Congo;
again, all without complications.[5] It is possible Koprowski's work in a commercial environment limited his visibility among more academic institutions
or laboratories. Likewise, his trials were probably not sufficiently acceptable

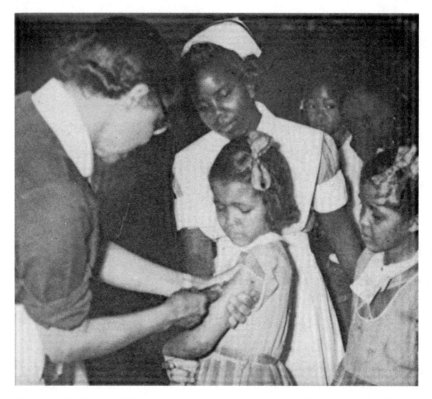

Figure 59. Children in Macon County receiving inoculations. (Courtesy of the Tuskegee University Archives)

for validation.[6] Although not directly associated with the work at Tuskegee, Koprowski's techniques were not conducted under as strict controls as that of the NFIP. Tuskegee's scientists and technicians were bound by stringent guidelines that ensured the quality of their outcomes.

Salk's primary competitor for the completion of a preventative for polio was Dr. Albert Sabin. The acrimonious debate between Salk and Sabin has been characterized as "anything but academic."[7] The animosity between the two was exacerbated by the constant debate among adherents of the respective methods of delivery. Those affiliated with Sabin argued his vaccine was "more effective, so it would virtually always trigger the desired defensive response, while Salk's supporters argued it put children at risk of contracting the disease through the vaccination."[8] Also, Salk's vaccine was introduced six years before Sabin's, creating a professional jealousy between the two. This jealousy led to verbal attacks by Sabin at various national meetings, prompting one of his colleagues to note about him: "he deserves a comeuppance."[9] The controversy continued between their colleagues and other health officials long after their deaths.[10]

It is interesting to note the Sabin vaccine had for thirty years become the norm in the United States.[11] The vaccine was taken orally on a sugar cube, in a bonbon, or mixed with syrup. The argument continued that the Sabin vaccine was economical, "easy to administer, immunizes swiftly, protects thoroughly, and provides 'near-immunity.'"[12] The Salk vaccine likewise had its champions and was deemed equally effective because it was safe for those with compromised (weakened) immune systems.[13]

Salk after the Vaccine

After the release of his vaccine, Salk's passion turned from the poliovirus to developing an independent research community devoted to biological research and studies, including immunology, autoimmune diseases, cancers, and other viruses such as Human Immunodeficiency Virus (HIV) and multiple sclerosis. Located in San Diego, California, the Salk Institute (built in 1967) occupies 27 acres and has sixty-one faculty members and a scientific staff of more than 850. The various laboratories house researchers working on an assortment of diseases from birth defects to Alzheimer's, Parkinson's, and AIDS. Salk became an accomplished author and died at age 80 on June 23, 1995. His three sons followed him into medicine, with Peter Salk dedicated to developing immune-based therapeutic vaccines for HIV and AIDS. Jonas Salk's memorial at the institute epitomizes his personal life and accomplishments. It reads: "Hope lies in dreams, in imagination and in the courage of those who dare to make dreams into reality."[14]

The NFIP and Tuskegee

The NFIP's dedication to working with Tuskegee is evident in how much was spent from 1939 to 1951. Not only did they support the building of the Infantile Paralysis wing of the John A. Andrew Memorial Hospital in 1939–1940 but also they provided a scholarship for nurses, established a brace shop and trained the brace-maker, assisted with operating funds for the Infantile Paralysis facility, and provided important funding for the nursing school. All of this amounted to $1,641,225.00, a very substantial sum at the time. Unfortunately, the March of Dimes does not have complete records or reports concerning the amount of money spent at Tuskegee during the Salk Vaccine Trials.[15] There is no doubt the amount was substantial. There is nothing nefarious about this; funds transferred between the NFIP and its grantees was accomplished on an as-needed basis. The NFIP did everything they could to keep the project solvent. In a letter between the directors of the NFIP and GWCRF, Weaver assured Brown, "assuming a reasonable effort on the part of the Institute, there would be no financial loss to you, irrespective of the result of this venture."[16]

By 1963, the NFIP had spent an additional $1,716,400.00 with $1,247,161.00 allocated directly to the Infantile Paralysis center.[17] Even though the vaccine was approved by 1955 and incidences of polio were on the decline, there were still patients needing medical assistance. The NFIP remained dedicated to helping all, whether black or white, who continued to bear the effects of the disease. After the Salk vaccine proved successful and the incidents of polio began to substantially wane, the NFIP had to refocus their mission statement.

Due to its previous endeavors toward seeking a preventative for infantile paralysis, the NFIP had expended most of its financial reserves. The success of the Salk and later Sabin vaccines emphasized the need for an organization like the NFIP. Their infrastructure included medical personnel, health educators, marketing and fund-raising professionals, and competent administrators that could accomplish the seemingly impossible. Now, with success in hand, they turned their attention toward helping "moms have full-term pregnancies and healthy babies."[18] They still utilize their resources by offering "information and comfort to families" and by researching "the problems that threaten our babies."[19]

The GWCRF Since 1955

Concurrent with the work on the Salk vaccine project, the GWCRF (now called the Carver Foundation) worked on perfecting its processes and procedures for mass producing and distributing the HeLa cell culture to other research laboratories. This work was projected to include other cell lines, making the work at Tuskegee laboratories more self-sustaining after the Salk vaccine trials were completed. However, this was not all the Carver Foundation was working on. Their work would prove to be wide ranging and important, with support coming from a variety of individuals (figure 60).

From its opening, scientists, many of whom had PhDs,[20] worked with such enigmatic problems as determining the best dietary intakes by human beings for optimal nutrition, to assessing the viability of kudzu as a partial feed and as a means of controlling erosion. Papers were presented at prestigious organizations such as the American Institute of Biological Sciences at Cornell University and to the Federation of American Societies for Experimental Biology in Chicago, Illinois. While initially formal instruction did not extend beyond the Master of Science degree, the Carver Foundation provided educational experiences to many young black scientists who had already received an advanced degree. They were employed as full-time research assistants and given

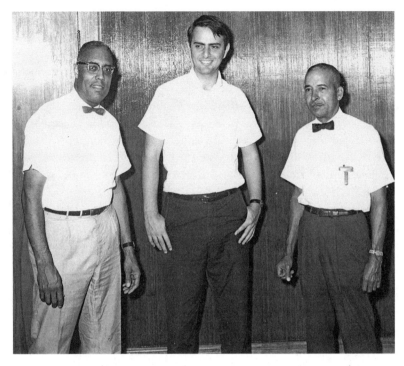

Figure 60. (*Right to left*) Dr. Russell Brown, director of the Carver Research Foundation; preeminent American scientist Carl Sagan; and Dr. James Henderson. assistant to Dr. Brown on the HeLa Cell Project. (Courtesy of the Tuskegee University Archives)

faculty status at Tuskegee University during the period of sponsored research, but equally valuable is the research experience they received. A number of these students went on to receive their PhDs in important fields such as agronomy, animal husbandry, chemistry (including organic and physical biochemistry), and foods and nutrition. Seeking to provide well-trained scientists with instructional experience was an essential part of their research program.

During the period from 1951 to 1952, the Carver Foundation received grants and contracts from at least twelve organizations other than the NFIP, including the National Institutes of Health (US Department of Public Health), International Minerals and Chemical Corporation, and the Upjohn Company. By the next year, they had received almost twice as many grants, and by 1982 they had received 77 grant or contracts from diverse groups such as NASA, Lilly Endowment, General Mills, Merck Company, and Dow Chemical. By 1984, the Carver Foundation had expanded its role to include: "providing the necessary quality control and evaluation of research being conducted by Tuskegee

University faculty and staff; and to maintain research facilities for the research being conducted by the Carver Research Foundation (CRF) staff."[21]

It had initially been planned that as soon as the evaluation of the Salk vaccine was completed, the Carver Foundation would continue to produce the "HeLa cell cultures in quantity for virus isolations and antibody titrations."[22] This commercial venture was strictly to support the foundation for years to come. The NFIP, in a letter from Dr. Henry W. Kumm to Dr. Thomas M. Rivers, reiterated their initial agreement with Tuskegee by noting: "It had been planned that as soon as this operation was proceeding in a satisfactory manner, direct support from the NFIP would terminate."[23] From 1955 onward, the Tuskegee Laboratories were to be self-sufficient. By 1956, one year after the evaluations, the foundation had incurred a $10,000 deficit, prompting the NFIP to cease underwriting the losses that were incurred. Further reasons for not supporting the work were succinctly stated by Basil O'Connor: "At the time the venture started, HeLa cell cultures were in great demand and we hoped that you would eventually be able to carry on the work at a profit. Since then, however, it has been shown that many of the newly discovered viruses will not grow on HeLa cell cultures. Consequently, many workers are using monkey kidney tissue cultures instead of HeLa cell cultures. In addition to this, commercial organizations are now supplying to laboratories cell cultures of many types."[24] Aware of this situation, the Tuskegee laboratories "communicated with 60 laboratories concerning future purchase of cultures and the replies received" indicated they could "sell about 1,000 tube cultures per week and not more than 10 bottle cultures per week."[25] Correspondence indicates the Carver Foundation was making a concerted effort to push their product to as many companies as possible.[26] In fact, from September to October 1954, sales of HeLa cell cultures were brisk, with 365 tubes and 15 bottles sold.[27]

It is apparent that other factors were keeping the CRF from succeeding. In a letter from Kumm to O'Connor, Kumm stated "because of the development of the Salk color test using trypsinized monkey kidney cells, the production capacity of the Tuskegee Laboratory was never used in full, even during the vaccine field trial."[28] Tuskegee's work with the HeLa cell cultures came to an end by 1956.

Dr. Timothy Turner,[29] a scientist at the CRF, writing in *The Journal of Health Care for the Poor and Underserved*, further explains: "In 1954, Microbiological Associates, Inc. copied the successful template designed at Tuskegee University's Carver Research Foundation," and "this template was used to set up a large-scale cell culture factory in a former Fritos factory in Bethesda, Maryland, to begin mass-producing HeLa cells for global distribution, simultaneously ushering in a multibillion-dollar industry for the selling of biomedical specimens."[30] Tuskegee's lab was small, not capable of sustaining large scale production and distribution. The CRF decided that competing with commercial producers like Microbiological Associates was not in their strategic plan for the future.

It is unclear whether, at the time, Tuskegee's scientists were aware of the origins of the HeLa cells with which they were working.[31] It is ironic that the very cells that were taken from an African American named Henrietta Lacks without her permission or compensation were later used for profit by a historically black university. Furthermore, it is also important to reiterate that her cells were used for one of the most important scientifically beneficial research projects of all time. The Salk vaccine field trials and subsequent inoculations benefited everyone, regardless of race or color. It is significant to note, while the situation concerning Lacks and the HeLa cell was not optimal, something incredibly advantageous came out of it for the whole world.

The Salk vaccine given in the 1950s had not been without controversy. Shortly after the vaccine was first delivered for inoculation (after the trial had ended), people in California and Idaho had "developed paralysis in the arm or leg where the vaccine was injected."[32] Due to changes in production techniques and procedures for producing the vaccine that deviated from those utilized in the field trials, 204 cases of poliomyelitis were eventually reported. The contamination was traced to Cutter Laboratories[33] of Berkeley, California, and possibly other laboratories, prompting Surgeon General Leonard Scheele to stop inoculations for approximately one week, from May 7 to May 13, 1955. Parke-Davis, one of the original testing laboratories, was allowed to resume producing the vaccine, but with more stringent quality control measures.

In 1960, when the Simian Virus, also known as SV40,[34] was first isolated and identified, it was discovered that it also existed in the current polio vaccine. The virus had been associated with certain types of cancer in humans, although it was unclear whether the virus caused them. From 1955 to 1963, approximately 98 million Americans received dosages that could have had some portion of the SV40 virus. It appears the virus was found only in the injected form of the polio vaccine. Since 1963, evidence suggests polio vaccines no longer contained SV40. Unfortunately, modern research techniques cannot re-create the events that happened over fifty years ago. Therefore, it is impossible to determine whether SV40 contributed to cancer in anyone.[35]

Within two years after the release of the Salk vaccine and the beginning of inoculations, Tuskegee laboratories became a "nationwide source for the supply of animal cell cultures."[36] In fact, they used other human cell cultures such as "H.E. p#2 strain from metastatic carcinoma of the larynx . . . cell strains from normal human conjunctiva, liver and appendix."[37] They even continued work with the HeLa cell culture. Under a grant from the National Institutes of Health (NIH), the laboratories reported "over a period of five years in our laboratory there has been no evidence of change in character of the strain HeLa when the medium contained 40 percent or more of human serum."[38] The methods, procedures, and quality control learned during the NFIP Salk vaccine trials propelled Tuskegee's Carver Foundation into national prominence.

By 1959, the CRF was designated a repository of mammalian cells by the National Cancer Institute and NIH. Its scientists worked to provide cells to "many laboratories in the United States and in foreign countries by supplying reference or seed cultures for use in research."[39] The objectives of the laboratories continued to morph and evolve to "the maintenance of reference cultures and the study of the characteristics of the individual cell strains."[40] This led to an increase, by 1960, of forty cell strains within its repository, and "five hundred starter cultures were distributed to other investigators during the past two years."[41]

Other innovations at the time overshadow the important work of the CRF. During the 1950s, new medical procedures, methods, tools, and medicines abounded throughout the nation. By 1951, image-analyzing microscopy was developed and initiated. In 1953, the first successful open-heart surgery was performed (using a heart-lung machine developed by John Gibbon Jr.), and prescription and nonprescription drugs were finally legally distinguished from one another. In the same year, James Watson and Francis Crick discovered the structure of the genetic material of DNA. In 1954, Texas Instruments created silicon transistors, and in 1958, the integrated circuit, greatly increasing the capabilities of the computer. By 1960, more successful and useful drugs had been developed such as isoniazid (a compound that when mixed with streptomycin provides an effective anti-tuberculosis drug) and Thorazine, an antipsychotic drug.

Alternatively, within this important decade, the three-dimensional structure of hemoglobin was determined, ultimately linking protein sequences that allowed scientists to apply specific targeting for physiological research and drug discovery. Much of this research and development can be traced to procedures and policies developed during the Salk vaccine field trial and the work at Tuskegee. Specifically, the work accomplished by the CRF provided needed information relative to research requiring in vitro[42] cell culture usage.[43]

Unfortunately, the work at Tuskegee and the CRF was often overlooked, with more prestigious schools claiming the notoriety for developing such pioneering research. This was contrary to a report titled "New Biological Assembly Lines," published in *MOSAIC*, November–December 1978, "describing large-scale production of HeLa cells by the Cell Culture Center, University of Alabama at Birmingham (UAB), which has been made available to other research laboratories. There was no mention of the work done at Tuskegee, which had been publicized extensively during the decade of the 1950s. It is interesting also that the Cell Culture Center is sponsored by the National Science Foundation, as is a similar cell culture center at Massachusetts Institute of Technology. The report implies that the UAB project was a pioneering venture."[44]

Obviously, UAB did not exercise due diligence in their search for further information regarding in vitro cell culture, especially at Tuskegee. Several national newspapers carried information about Tuskegee's work with the NFIP field trials for the Salk vaccine, providing detailed information about new techniques with cell cultures. This is confirmed in an article dated 1956, which stated "that the HeLa cell was first mass-produced and shipped at Tuskegee Institute under NFIP sponsorship."[45] In order for the cells to be mass-produced and successfully shipped, they required some method to keep them alive.

Although most of the medical breakthroughs that occurred in the 1950s happened elsewhere, the CRF was instrumental in developing new equipment and techniques still in use today. In 1965, Dr. Russell Brown, Karl H. Bloss and Louise H. Beacham published a paperntitled "Vial Impinger for Storage of Mammalian Cells and Sampling of Viral Agents in Aerosols,"[46] touting the development of a system for the detection of viral agents in aerosols. The apparatus was used to impinge, or force, "aerosol upon a culture of mammalian cells preserved in the impinger vessel by liquid nitrogen refrigeration."[47] This process did not damage the cells or impede the rate of cell proliferation after thawing had occurred. Furthermore, the development of the impinger was in response to the large quantity of cells held inside the repository and the need to freeze cell lines for future work. By 1960, the American Type Culture Repository (ATCC) was established by the National Cancer Institute and samples of Tuskegee's cells were provided for inclusion. It then became evident the role of the experimental repository program at Tuskegee had served its original purpose.[48]

Carver's vision had come to fruition. The CRF was intended to be an organization that provided "facilities and a measure of support for young Negroes engaged in advanced scientific research."[49] Carver saw it as a place where black students had an opportunity to unlock "the mysteries of the universe in order to improve the quality of life for everyone, particularly the poor and underprivileged."[50] That is exactly what the CRF did; it provided black scientists the opportunity to show they, too, could compete with their white counterparts, while achieving loftier goals which contributed to the betterment of all of mankind.

The NFIP's New Vision

After the success of the Salk vaccine and subsequent Sabin vaccine, the NFIP, now called the March of Dimes, had accomplished their initial research goal. Their continued thrust refocused on childhood diseases, prenatal care, and birth defects. As of 1970, they broadened their vision to include improving birth results by incorporating perspectives in perinatal health, which meant appropriately considering the health of all pregnant women and babies in an attempt to minimize or eliminate birth defects, infant mortality, and low-birthweight babies. March of Dimes grants and funding "for medical services shifted to neonatal intensive care, genetic counseling, and perinatal networks; and funds for statewide networks of intensive care for high-risk infants led in turn to grants for the training of medical professionals in prenatal evaluation and care of high-risk pregnancies."[51] The March of Dimes' new slogan "Be Good to Your Baby before It Is Born" exemplified their new philosophy. This was to be accomplished through "proactive prenatal care in programs such as Operation Stork and Stork's Nest to educate women about healthy pregnancy at the community level."[52]

The March of Dimes also turned its attention to debilitating and often deadly maladies such as HIV/AIDS and substance abuse. The challenges of both HIV/AIDS and substance abuse began to reach cataclysmic proportions in the 1980s, and the March of Dimes addressed such problems wherever they impacted the health of mothers and babies.[53] They articulated these breakthroughs into wide-ranging public health messages about avoiding alcohol during pregnancy and proper nutrition for both expectant mothers and newborn babies. Its campaigns were directed to everyone, no matter their race, creed, religion, or social standing.

During the 1950s and 1960s, the March of Dimes had a strong advocate within the black community in Charles Bynum. After the completion of the licensing of the Salk and Sabin vaccines, Bynum became concerned with the declining membership and participation of African Americans as the March of Dimes ceased granting to all institutions. In an attempt to maintain the support of both black individuals and institutions, Bynum argued in 1963 "that future materials [should] reflect a gradually accelerated project of awareness of the increased importance of all market publics."[54] This, he contended, could only be accomplished through the implementation of black inclusion in all aspects of the March of Dimes' work and "increased use of black subject matter in the foundation's national advertising and publicity efforts."[55] The strategy worked, and the March of Dimes flourished under the banner of racial equality during a time of intense racial turmoil.

The relationship between Tuskegee and the March of Dimes was not just any partnership. Edith Powell wrote in her book *A Black Oasis: Tuskegee Institute's Fight Against Infantile Paralysis, 1941–1975*, "It was a profound partnership, unshakeable and lasting for many years. There were many facets which continue to this day. It enabled deep friendships, built trusts, permitted outstanding accomplishments and created wealth. Not dollars, but education for hundreds who were fortunate recipients of this relationship."[56]

Final Thoughts

Tuskegee's first five administrations were the catalysts for ongoing endeavors in health care-related fields. Each one brought a unique perspective that dove tailed into the previous president's work. The key to all of this was financial support. Without it, health-care and/or scientific research at Tuskegee faltered or even halted. Tuskegee, being a small school averaging three thousand students, was unable to absorb consistently large deficits. Some programs were able to be self supportive through grants or government-related funds. The CRF continued to receive some funding, but it was minimal at best.[57]

The CRF's work with the HeLa cell during the field trial and afterward would not have been successful without the support of the administration of Dr. Luther H, Foster, the fourth president of Tuskegee University. Beyond his ongoing support of the work at the CRF, Foster is credited with adding classes (1958–1959) in public health and mental health to the nursing curriculum. He further instigated an agreement between the university and the Veterans Administration (1957–1958), in which graduates of the Department of Physical Education's Corrective Therapy Program were immediately hired to full-time positions. Foster also increased support to the department of hospital dietetics and later established the allied health program.[58] All of this was in response to the respect Tuskegee graduates had as scientists and health-care professionals.

During the term of Tuskegee's fifth president Dr. Benjamin F. Payton, the university was forced to reexamine its role in health care, especially within the local community. Over the course of a decade, the John A. Andrew Memorial Hospital had continued to lose money. Coupled with a declining base of patients and the rising cost of medical supplies and personnel, the hospital had lost more than eight million dollars, with its final year (1986–1987) of operation seeing a deficit of one million. When it closed on October 1, 1987, Payton lamented, "For more than 75 years it (i.e., the hospital) had provided health care for blacks not only in Macon County, but in many other communities in the State. Especially in earlier years when blacks were not afforded equal access to Alabama health care facilities, this hospital filled an unmet need for its clientele. In those times, also, an important part of Tuskegee's mission was to provide assistance and services to Blacks when these were not available otherwise. However, by 1987, we could no longer sacrifice the quality of our educational programs to accommodate a medical care facility for the poor."[59]

The reason the hospital closed was purely a financial decision. The Board of Trustees could no longer afford to back the rising debts incurred by the hospital, which had been hemorrhaging money for several years."[60] Additionally, the financial problems of the hospital were further impacted as a result of integration. Integration contributed to the decline of the hospital, since patients could now choose to go to other medical facilities for a wider range of services or, as with the staff and physicians, increased opportunities. The John A. Andrew Memorial Hospital could no longer compete with these institutions, and Tuskegee University no longer felt it was feasible to keep it open.

The role of Tuskegee in health care, especially amongst black patients cannot be overemphasized. Booker T. Washington's notion of a healthy "head, hand and heart" permeated every aspect of the school's teaching and training for years to come. During the administrations of each of its first four presidents, Tuskegee made significant inroads into health care-related themes for black people, not only in rural Alabama but throughout the world. The institution's cooperation to provide "blood serum from a number of students," in 1957, "for a study on human gamma globulin to be used to cure rabies," in conjunction with "the Population Council to provide patients for a study on intrauterine devices (IUDS)" in 1963 underscores its place in health-care research.[61] Importantly, it was not only black citizens who benefited from the work, but all races. Nowhere was this more evident than in the creation of the Salk vaccine.

Imagine, in the 1950s, black scientists and researchers working toward the development of a vaccine that helped millions of Americans, most of them white. There have been many times black and white people have worked together for the common good of all mankind. The efforts of the NFIP and Tuskegee University's staff working together to overcome the deadly disease of polio are but one example of such cooperation. Sadly, the negative is often emphasized without realizing the positive. How different the world might be if we worked equally hard on all social and civic problems. There have been substantial gains made during the last century, and while there is no doubt that institutional and scientific racism have declined, there is still much more to be accomplished.

After the completion of the NFIP's field trial during the late 1950s and 1960s, political elevation of black citizens ensued at a rapid rate. Large numbers of African Americans began to take a variety of actions to do away with segregation, legal discrimination, and political disenfranchisement. Rosa Parks's 1955 refusal to relinquish her seat to a white man on a bus in Montgomery, Alabama, led to the Montgomery Bus Boycott. This event has been declared as the beginning of the modern civil rights movement, which successfully drew the attention of the national media to the plight of African Americans in Alabama and beyond. Events such as popular outrage over poll taxes and literacy tests (that prevented black and poor people from voting in the Southeast), sit-in demonstrations around the nation, Freedom Rides, and the dramatic march from Selma to Montgomery by Dr. Martin Luther King Jr. and other protesters in the spring of 1965 were further accompanied by extensive media coverage. Public opinion escalated dramatically toward a resolution of these issues. These events combined to force President Lyndon Johnson's administration into signing the Voting Rights Act of 1965.[62] It has been noted that legal segregation and black disenfranchisement ended in this country largely due to events that occurred in Alabama's Black Belt region,[63] of which Tuskegee played an integral part. Finally, while all of this was occurring, the Salk vaccine trials were completed and everyone, black and white, began to benefit from the preventative established by the mutual efforts of scientists, black and white. That the triumph of the Salk vaccine trials occurred at the very beginning of the Second Reconstruction[64] is an example of the beneficent alignment of science and social change that eventually remade the South and the nation.

Tuskegee University's legacy is more than Booker T. Washington, George Washington Carver, the Tuskegee Airmen, and the syphilis study; it is men and women working toward the betterment of society. From the Jesup Wagon to the Carver Research Foundation, Tuskegee has been involved with health-related issues for the underserved community of the South. All of this was accomplished through education and services to all, regardless of race. What mattered was helping those who were in need. Maybe this is what drew Basil O'Connor, the NFIP, and others to Tuskegee when they could have gone elsewhere.

The successes of Tuskegee could not have been accomplished without the financial aid and service of those white men and women who believed in the mission of Tuskegee. Although few, they were not bound by the constraints of segregation and racism. It is amazing what can be accomplished when men and women look beyond the color of one's skin and see the possibilities, no matter how impossible they may seem.

While there is still significant room for improvement, much has changed over the past fifty years. People have changed, laws have changed, and institutions have changed toward better black and white relations. Dialogue driven by the evolution of a nation and its people from abject segregation toward improved acceptance and toleration is now the conventional norm. But, with all that has been accomplished in race relations, how far have we come? When the vaccine was first given, one must wonder how many would have taken it if they had known of its origins with an underprivileged black woman by the name of Henrietta Lacks. Additionally, would they have taken the vaccine if they had known a portion of the work originated at a historically black college, Tuskegee University?

Epilogue

In 2011, Tuskegee University (the Carver Research Foundation), the More-house School of Medicine, and the University of Alabama at Birmingham (UAB) Comprehensive Cancer Center entered into research collaboration designed to attack disparate rates of cancer mortality among black people. This research tri-angle is the result of an effort of the National Cancer Institute (NCI), which pairs federally designated comprehensive cancer centers such as UAB and in-stitutions of higher learning that historically serve minorities (HBCUs). The primary objectives "are to maintain progress in establishing productive cancer research programs at MSM and TU, to persist in developing a pipeline of pro-spective minority investigators at TU and further expand cancer disparity re-search at UABCCC."[1]

Writing in a pamphlet for an exhibit at the Tuskegee University Legacy Museum, Curator Jontyle Robinon emphasized this program by noting: "The partnership's necessity and importance of addressing ethical issues such as the ones raised by Johns Hopkins University Hospital's treatment of Lacks and her family by hospital staff and doctors cannot be overstated." She goes on to express its further importance to "help researchers: to anticipate the kind of ethical issues their research might raise, to examine these issues, and to criti-cally reflect on how they plan to resolve them."[2] The bioethical implications of what transpired at Johns Hopkins; Macon County, Alabama (the USPHSSS);[3] and other locations are important enough to warrant greater emphasis in medi-cine, political theory, and law. Just as racial discrimination and segregation must come to an end through concerted efforts by the international community, established boundaries of medical ethics must be adhered to by all.

Appendix 1

African American March of Dimes Poster Children (1947–1960)

Year	Name	Hometown	Poster Slogan	Photo#
1947	Rita Reed	Blue Island, IL	Your Dimes Helped Me	199
1948	Joe Willie Brown	Chicago, IL	Please! Join the MOD	200A
1949	Rose Marie Waters	Washington, DC	Look! I can walk again	98
1950	Roxie Louise Prince	Americus, GA	I'm Winning Because of You	201A
1951	Joya Moore	Montgomery, AL	Lend me a hand	50-2290
1952	Emma Pearl Berry	Raymond, MS	Give Voluntarily-Join MOD	51-654A
1953	Randy Donoho	Detroit, MI	You can help, too!	52-2098
1954	Cynthia Musgrove	Pompano Beach, FL	Help Now! Reaseach will win	53-783
1955	James Clark Allen	Tyler, TX	Fight Polio!	54-1639
1956	Phyllis Townsend	Los Angeles, CA	Help me, too	55-2527
1957	Calvin Mayfield	Cleveland, OH	Remember Me	56-2206
1958	Eloise Sturgis	Augusta, GA	Join the MOD-They need YOU!	57-1653
1959	Wade Irby	Washington, DC	Give New Hope! Polio/Virus	58-1416
	Sheila Fleming	Washington, DC	Diseases/Arthritis/Birth Defects	
1960	Darrell Atkins	Brooklyn, NY	Prevent Crippling Diseases/ Birth Defects/Arthritis/Polio	59-2128

December 28, 2004/David Rose/March of Dimes Archives

Appendix 2

Procedures for Inoculations

The inoculums were received in packages of six vials each, three containing 10 cc. of vaccine, and three containing the same amount of placebo, the quantity required for the three injections of twenty children. The method of packaging and the code system were devised to ensure that lot and sub-lot numbers (vaccine or control solution) could be identified without revealing the code. This procedure also assured that equal quantities in each inoculation clinic without identification of the substance in the field. It also provided a means of making sure that each subject received three successive injections of the same lot of material.

The classroom groups of the first, second, and third grades of a participating school constituted the basic clinic unit and remained so through the three inoculations. The following plan of procedure was outlined in the *Manual of Suggested Procedures*.

As each class appears at the clinic, the teacher will accompany each child into the clinic room in alphabetical order. (The Vaccination Records forms should also be in alphabetical order, as should the listing of children's names on the Registration Schedule, both previously prepared from the forms signed by the parents and the teacher's classroom roll.) In the placebo control areas it will be essential that classrooms attending a given clinic follow each other in the same sequence in succeeding clinics.

As the child enters the room, the recorder should verify with the teacher the identification of the child, and place that child's Vaccination Record on the table before her. The physician should call out to the recorder the lot number of the vaccine to be given to that child. The recorder should record the lot number on the Vaccination Record. Having done so, she should repeat the lot number so that the physician can verify her recording. The month and day of vaccination should then be recorded on the Registration Schedule.

. . . The physician will then give the vaccine in the left triceps muscle. (If for some special reason another site of inoculation is used, notation indicating the actual site should be made under "Remarks" on the Vaccination Record.)

The dose of material given should be accurately measured as 1 cc. The recommended procedure is to fill each syringe to the 5cc. mark, using 1 cc. for each of 5 children, changing the needle each time . . . accurate measurement of dosage is essential, since it is planned to inject 10 children from each vial.

A second sterile syringe was used to remove from the vial the remaining 5 cc. which was then administered to five additional children.

The 10 cc. of material from the first of a pair of vials, bearing one lot number, was used to inoculate the first ten children listed on the Registration Schedule of a given class. The second 10 cc. vial bearing the other lot number and containing the other inoculums was used for the next ten children. The remaining four vials in the package were set aside to be used in similar fashion for the second and third injections of the same children. Before returning these vials to the refrigerator, however, the recorder entered the name of the school, the grade, and the Registration Schedule number on the end label on the package.

At the second series of inoculations (V-Day plus one week), children were arranged in the same sequence within classes and in class order as at the time of the first inoculation. Material from the second pair of vials was used making sure that the number of the lot given to each child matched the code shown on his Vaccination Record to have been used for the previous injection.

The package of material was opened as the designated group of children approached the physician's station, and when the group had received the specified material, the vials were returned to the package which was then removed to prevent use in the wrong group of children and prepared for storage until the next scheduled clinic.

. . . If a child whose parents requested vaccination was not present for the first injection, he received no injection at any subsequent time. On the other hand, every effort was made to continue inoculations in those who received the first but were absent at the time of the second or third clinics. To accomplish this, make-up clinics were organized, usually at a central location.

. . . Children were give a Polio Volunteer button from the National Foundation after the first inoculation . . . and a Polio Pioneer Award card was given to all children who completed the full series of three inoculations . . . Special recognition was also given to those who participated in the serological studies by donating specimens of blood. The distribution of these awards was ordinarily made at a ceremony at the end of the vaccination program and after the second specimens of blood has been procured.

Authors' Note: The Manual of Suggested Procedures for the Conduct of the Vaccine Field Trial in 1954 (White Plains, NY: National Foundation for Infantile Paralysis, 1953); taken from the Final Report, 55. In a memorandum (No. 1) from the Vaccine Evaluation Center, dated April 14, 1954, State and Local Health Officers were instructed, "Uniformity of procedure in the field operations is of greatest importance in order to reduce error and confusion in the data as well as to ensure that cases from the study groups will be detected promptly, and that clinical, epidemiological and laboratory investigations can be instituted at the appropriate times. Procedures, which it is hoped will be followed, have been recommended with the objective of attaining the essential uniformity."

Appendix 3

HeLa Production Personnel at Tuskegee

Administrative

R. W. Brown, Director
R. J. Harris, Expediter
Alma R. Hunter, Stenographer

Tissue Culture Technicians

Gloria Mobiley, Laboratory Supervisor
Evelyn Carmon
Angela DuBose
Caselle C. Knox II
Jeanne M. Walton
Arnette Matchett
Mildred R. Forte
Lessie Ducksworth
Corine Milburn
Joyce Perry
Louise Beacham

Laboratory Helpers

James C. Harris, Supervisor
Carl W. Cotton
Leon B. Hill
Frederick Ratcliff
Clarence L. Mason
George J. Esther

Shipping Clerks

Curtis Turner
Charles W. Hayden

Lemuel Locklair
Mable J. Woods

Student Helpers

Mary Baxter
Blanchard Robinson
Pauline Jenkins
Joseph Jackson
Isaac Bembry
Melvin Fussel
Royland Jones
Roscoe Bell

Appendix 4

*NFIP Grantee Laboratories Receiving HeLa Cultures
from Tuskegee, 1953–1955*

Laboratory	Scientist(s)
*School of Hygiene & Public Health The Johns Hopkins University Baltimore, MD	David Bodian Howard A. Howe
School of Public Health University of Michigan Ann Arbor, MI	Gordon C. Brown Donald E. Craig
Laboratories of the Department of Health Albany, NY	Gilbert Dalidorf Johan Winsser
Children's Hospital Boston, MA	John F. Enders Sydney Kibrick
Department of Bacteriology & Immunology University of North Dakota Grand Forks, ND	Robert G. Fischer
School of Medicine Tulane University New Orleans, LA	John P. Fox Louis Potash
School of Medicine University of Oregon Portland, OR	Arthur W. Frisch

Department of Bacteriology   Louis P. Gebhardt
University of Utah College of Medicine
Salt Lake City, UT

*College of Medicine   Seymore S. Kalter
State University of New York
Syracuse, NY

Department of Bacteriology   David T. Karzon
University of Buffalo Medical School
Buffalo, NY

Department of Health, Education, & Welfare   Carl L. Larson
Rocky Mountain Laboratory
Hamilton, MT

Viral & Rickettsial Disease Laboratory   Edwin H. Lennette
Berkeley, CA

Microbiological Associates   M. R. Hilleman
Bethesda, MD

School of Medicine   Joseph L. Melnick
Yale University
New Haven, CT

Department of Infectious Diseases   Aaron F. Rasmussen
University of California Medical Center
Los Angeles, CA

*Department of Bacteriology   Robert Rustigian
University of Chicago
Chicago, IL

Communicable Disease Center   Morris Schaeffer
Viral and Rickettsial Laboratories   Alan Bernstein
Montgomery, AL

*Division of Laboratories   Howard J. Shaughnessy
Department of Public Health
Chicago, IL

*School of Medicine University of Louisville Louisville KY	Alex J. Steigman Murray M. Lipton
Department of Bacteriology & Immunology University of Minnesota Minneapolis, MN	Jerome T. Syverton
*Department of Pediatrics Medical Center University of Kansas Kansas City, KS	Herbert A. Wenner
Department of Bacteriology University of Manitoba Winnipeg, Canada	J. C. Wilt
Connaught Medical Research Laboratories University of Toronto Toronto, Canada	R. D. Defries D. R. E. MacLeod

*Indicates laboratories that originally planned to use monkey kidney cells in lieu of HeLa cell cultures.

Appendix 5

Cell Strains in the Experimental Cell Repository at Tuskegee University from 1955 to 1961

Cell No.	Designation	Subsequent ACC No.
1	HeLa (Gey) Original*	CCL-2
2	HeLa (Gey) Clone	S-1*
3	HeLa (Gey) S-3*	CCL-2.2
4	HeLa (Gey) S3–9*	——
5	Human Appendix (Chang) Clone A-1*	——
6	Human Conjunctiva (Chang) Clone C-1 (Puck)*#	CCL-20.2
7	HeLa (Gey) D Line*	——
8	HeLa (Gey) X Line*	——
9	HEp #2 (Moore, Sabachewsky & Toolaa)*#	CCL-23
10	FL Human Amnion (Fogh & Lund)*#	CCL-62
11	HH Human Heart (Girardi)*#	——
12	KB Human carcinoma of the Nasopharynx (Eagle)*#	CCL-17
13	Monkey Kidney MS (Tytell)	——
14	Sarcoma 180, Mouse (Foley & Drolet)	CCL-8
15	Thymus, Human, Normal (Foley & Eagle)	——
16	"Walker" Human Nasal Polyp (Foley et al.)	——
17	"Wilms'-6", Human Tumor (Foley et al)	——
18	Erlich's Ascites	——
19	"Lymph Node," Human	——
20	Ependymoma, Human	——
21	Astrocytoma, Human	——
22	Melanoma, Cloudman	CCL-53.1
23	Strain L, NCTC 929	CCL-1
24	Strain L, NCTC 2071	CCL-1.1
25	Human Liver (Chang)#	CCL-13
26	J96 Monocytic Leukemia	——
27	J111 Granulocytic Leukemia	——
28	MDBK Bovine Kidney, Normal (Madin & Darby)	CCL-22
29	MDCK Canine Kidney (Madin & Darby)	CCL-34

*First twelve strains in 1955.
#Subsequently shown to have HeLa markers.

Notes

Introduction

Epigraph. G. Lake Imes, *The Philosophies of Booker T. Washington* (Tuskegee, AL: Tuskegee Institute Press, 1941), 10.

1. Although referred to as Tuskegee Institute or Tuskegee Normal, the authors will use the current name, Tuskegee University, for all references.

2. Both of these began through the efforts of Booker T. Washington, the first principal at Tuskegee.

3. Authors have chosen to follow the *The Chicago Manual of Style* (sixteenth edition), which says, "Common designations of ethnic groups by color are usually lowercased unless a particular publisher or author prefers otherwise" (402). While the authors choose to use the term "black(s)" in lieu of African American(s) or Negro(es), all quotes will retain their original conventions.

4. They were, respectively, Alice Coachman and Nell Jackson.

5. Daniel "Chappie" James and Charles Gomillion.

6. Poliovirus is a member of the Picornaviridae family, a group of non-enveloped positive-strand RNA viruses.

7. Booker T. Washington, *Up From Slavery* (New York: Doubleday, Page and Company, 1901), 43.

8. The authors define the word "science" as "the concerted human effort to understand, or to understand better, the history of the natural world and how the natural world works, with observable physical evidence as the basis of that understanding. It is done through observation of natural phenomena, and/or through experimentation that tries to simulate natural processes under controlled conditions." Bruce Railsback, "What Is Science," accessed July, 27, 2016, http://www.gly.uga.edu/railsback/1122science2.html. Also, see: Edward O. Wilson, *Consilience: The Unity of Knowledge* (New York: Random House, 1999). For further information on the evolving definition of "science," see: Joel Isaac, *Working Knowledge: Making the Human Sciences from Parsons to Kuhn* (Cambridge, MA: Harvard University Press, 2012).

9. Information on the general history of the study (including Moton quotation) from: "U.S. Public Health Service Study at Tuskegee," Centers for Disease Control, https://www.cdc.gov/tuskegee/timeline.htm. Accessed on Septem-

ber 25, 2017. Although generally called the "Tuskegee syphilis study," the official name of the government's 1932–1972 study is the "The Study of Untreated Syphilis in the Male Negro in Macon County, Alabama." Susan Reverby, *Tuskegee's Truths: Rethinking the Tuskegee Syphilis Study* (Chapel Hill: University of North Carolina Press, 2000), 101. For more, see: Paul A. Lumbardo and Gregory M. Dorr, "Eugenics, Medical Education, and the Public Health Service: Another Perspective on the Tuskegee Syphilis Experiment," *Bulletin of the History of Medicine*, 80:2, summer 2006, 291–316.

10. Gloria A. Marshall, "Racial Classifications Popular and Scientific," *The "Racial" Economy of Science: Toward a Democratic Future*, ed. Sandra Harding (Bloomington: Indiana University Press, 1993).

11. Comte de Buffon is often credited with being the first to use the word race as a method to describe the variety of peoples throughout the world. Georges-Louis Leclerc, *Comte de Buffon, Natural History, General and Particular*, trans. William Smellie (1791; rpt. Bristol, UK: Thoemmes Press, 2000). M. F. Ashley Montagu, *Man's Most Dangerous Myth: The Fallacy of Race* (New York: Columbia University Press, 1942), 39.

12. Montagu, *Man's Most Dangerous Myth*, 37.

13. Also, see: A. C. Higgins, "Scientific Racism: A review of The Science and Politics of Racial Research by William H. Tucker," *Mathematicians of the African Diaspora* (Chicago: University of Illinois Press, 1994). Also, Gloria A. Marshall, "Racial Classifications Popular and Scientific," *The "Racial" Economy of Science: Toward a Democratic Future*, ed. Sandra Harding (Bloomington: Indiana University Press, 1993). For more information see: Theodore M. Porter, Dorothy Ross, eds., *The Cambridge History of Science: The Modern Social Sciences* (Cambridge, UK: Cambridge University Press, Vol. 7, 2003), 293: "Race has long played a powerful popular role in explaining social and cultural traits, often in ostensibly scientific terms"; Adam Kuper, Jessica Kuper, eds., "Racism," *The Social Science Encyclopedia* (1996), 716: "This [*scientific*] racism entailed the use of 'scientific techniques', to sanction the belief in European and American racial Superiority"; "Race, theories of," *Routledge Encyclopedia of Philosophy: Questions to Sociobiology* (1998), 18: "Its exponents [*of scientific racism*] tended to equate race with species and claimed that it constituted a scientific explanation of human history"; Paul A. Erickson and Liam D. Murphy, *A History of Anthropological Theory* (Toronto: UTP Higher Education, 2008), 152: "Scientific racism: Improper or incorrect science that actively or passively supports racism."

14. Reverby, *Tuskegee Truths*, 16.

15. Terry Jay Ellingson, *The Myth of the Noble Savage* (Oakland: University of California Press, 2001), 151: "In scientific racism, the racism was never very scientific; nor, it could at least be argued, was whatever met the qualifications of actual science ever very racist.

16. Arthur de Gobineau, *An Essay on the Inequality of the Human Races* (New York: G. P. Putnam and Sons, 1915) and Georges Vacher de Lapouge, C. Clossen, (1899), "Old and New Aspects of the Aryan Question," *The American Journal of Sociology 5* (3): 329–46.

17. William Z. Ripley. *The Races of Europe: A Sociological Study*, Lowell Institute Lectures (London: K. Paul Trench, Trubner & Co., Ltd., 1913). Also, see: E. Barkan, *The Retreat of Scientific Racism: Changing Concepts of Race in Britain and the United*

States Between the World Wars (Cambridge, UK: Cambridge University Press, 1992); W. Moore, "Red Pill Hangovers, Covert Racism, and the Sociological Machine," *American Sociological Association*, 42, 2013, 529–32. Moore, W, (2013).

18. Stephen J. Gould, "American Polygeny and Craniometry before Darwin," *The "Racial" Economy of Science: Toward a Democratic Future*, Sandra Harding, ed. (Bloomington: Indiana University Press, 1993), 87.

19. Ibid.

20. George O. Ferguson, *The Psychology of the Negro* (Westport, CT: Negro Universities Press, 1916).

21. Alexander Thomas & Samuel Sillen, *Racism and Psychiatry* (New York: Brunner/Mazel, Inc., 1972), 35.

22. Paul A. Lombardo and Gregory M. Dorr, "Eugenics, Medical Education, and the Public Health Service: Another Perspective on the Tuskegee Syphilis Experiment," *Bulletin of the History of Medicine*, 2006, 80:291–316. Eugenics utilized a technique called anthropometry as a means to show the differences between the races by measuring different parts of the body and comparing the findings in order to prove that they were "separated by hereditary differences." For further information see: Paul A. Lombardo, "Anthropometry, Race, and Eugenic Research: Measurements of Growing Negro Children at the Tuskegee Institute, 1932–1944." *The Uses of Humans in Experiment: Perspectives from the 17th to the 20th Century*, Ed. Erika Dyck and Larry Stewart (Boston: Brill Rodopi, 2016), 215.

23. For more information on eugenics, see: Frank Dikotter, "Race Culture: Recent Perspectives on the History of Eugenics," *The American Historical Review*, Vol. 103, No. 2 (Apr., 1998) and Edwin Black, *War Against the Weak: Eugenics and America's Campaign to Create a Master Race* (New York: Dialog Press, 2003).

24. Robert Bennett Bean, *The Races of Man: Differentiation and Dispersal of Man* (New York: University Society, 1932), 53.

25. W. B. Smith, *The Color Line* (Westport, CT: Negro Universities Press, 1969 [1905]), 187.

26. Charles Cerami, *Benjamin Banneker: Surveyor, Astronomer, Publisher, Patriot* (New York: John Wiley & Sons, Inc., 2002).

27. Ava Henry & Michael Williams, *Black Scientists and Inventors Book One* (London: BIS Enterprises Ltd., 2002).

28. Sarah Goode, *Inventors*, The Black Inventor On-Line Museum, 2011, Retrieved 8 March 2012.

29. Wini Warren, *Black Women Scientists in the United States*, (Bloomington: Indiana University Press, 2000).

30. W. E. B Du Bois, *Black Folk, Then and Now: An Essay in the History and Sociology of the Negro Race* (New York: H. Holt and Company, 1939), vii.

31. John P. Jackson, Jr. & Nadine M. Weidman. *Race, Racism, and Science: Social Impact and Interaction* (Santa Barbara, CA: ABC-CLIO, Inc., 2004), 129.

32. Ibid., 130.

33. Thomas & Sillen, *Racism and Psychiatry*, 32.

34. "Analyzing ethnic education policy-making in England and Wales," *Sheffield Online Papers in Social Research*, University of Sheffield, 12 (accessed June 20, 2006).

35. Maulana Karenga, *Introduction to Black Studies*, 3rd edition (Timbuktu, Mali: University of Sankore Press, 2002).

Chapter 1

Epigraph. *Selected Speeches of Booker T. Washington*, E. Davidson Washington, ed. (Garden City, New York: Doubleday, Doran and Company, Inc., 1932), 37.

1. Dana R. Chandler, "Tuskegee University," *The New Encyclopedia of Southern Culture, Volume 17, Education*, Clarence L. Mohr, ed. (Chapel Hill: University of North Carolina Press, 2011), 323.

2. For more information about Washington, see: *Up From Slavery* and Albon L Holsey, *Booker T. Washington's Own Story of His Life and Work* (Tuskegee, AL: Booker T. Washington, 1901).

3. The forerunner of the Tuskegee University Archives.

4. Washington, *Up From Slavery*, 54.

5. Booker T. Washington, *Southern Workman*, Vol. 10, No. 9, p. 94.

6. Additional information about the curriculum (*Tuskegee Institute Bulletins*) at Tuskegee can be found at the Tuskegee University Archives.

7. From here on referred to as the VA Hospital.

8. *The Tuskegee University Bulletin Courses and Programs: 2004–2006*, 410–11.

9. Since its inception in 1999, the Tuskegee University National Center for Bioethics in Research and Health Care has been committed to stimulating interest in and maintaining a national focus on the moral issues underlying biomedical research and medical treatment of African Americans and other underserved populations in this country.

10. Dr. Eugene Dibble, the medical director of the John A. Andrew Memorial Hospital, did participate in the study. Initially, he and then President Robert Moton "were assured that this was a research study to examine the necessity of treatment." Although the hospital was located on the grounds of Tuskegee University and they did receive funding from the university, it has not been shown that the administration knew of the study. Susan Reverby, in her book *Examining Tuskegee: The Infamous Syphilis Study and Its Legacy* (Chapel Hill: University of North Carolina Press, 2009), speaks of Dibble's culpability (see pages 152–66) while noting his "motives remain a mystery . . . it is clear that Dibble understood what the study was about and supported it until his death."

11. Health care at that time included a focus on education about nutrition and sanitation because students entered school with poor dietary and sanitary habits. Health care was about prevention of illness or disease.

12. Louis R. Harlan, ed., *The Booker T. Washington Papers*, Vol. 3, (Urbana: University of Illinois Press, 1974), 583–87.

13. *The Tuskegee University Bulletin Courses and Programs: 1881–1882*, 8.

14. Cornelius Nathaniel Dorsette, *Encyclopedia of Alabama*, accessed on May 11, 2015, http://www.encyclopediaofalabama.org/article/h-3282.

15. That is, with a college degree.

16. Booker T. Washington, "The Negro Doctor in the South," *The Independent*, July 11, 1907, 89.

17. Ibid.

18. John Kenney, writing about the status of "The Negro in the United States of America," notes: "Negro physicians and surgeons numbered 1,734 in the year 1900, and besides these there were 212 colored dentists and 200 pharmacists. While a few educated physicians and apothecaries, some of them slave-born, were practicing

among their people as early as the end of the eighteenth century; the majority of the Negro "doctors" consisted till far into the nineteenth century of "root doctors" who healed by spells and by practicing by superstition." Linda Kenney Miller, *The Negro in Medicine* (Marietta, GA: Harper House Publishers, 2008), 59–60.

19. Dorsette was appointed to Tuskegee's board of trustees where he served until his death.

20. "Black Hospital Movement in Alabama," *Encyclopedia of Alabama*, accessed May 12, 2015, http://www.encyclopediaofalabama.org/article/h-2410#sthash.QvjHnQ1M.dpuf. Dorsette was instrumental in starting an infirmary in Montgomery as early as 1890. The Hale Infirmary, the first such facility for black patients in Alabama, remained operational until 1958.

21. "The First Female Physician in Alabama," *Birmingham Medical News*, accessed May 12, 2015, http://www.birminghammedicalnews.com/news.php?viewStory =1530.

22. Ibid.

23. Before the Civil War, some white slave owners sought to tend illness and disease among their slaves with organized medical care. *Practical Rules for the Management and Medical Treatment of Negro Slaves in the Sugar Colonies* (London: J. Barfield, 1811). Later, in response to the medical needs of the newly freed slaves, white communities established segregated hospitals that were white owned and operated. Primarily located in the South, "these 'separate but equal' hospitals were often inadequate, provided substandard care, and rarely provided access for black physicians or nurses." "Opening Doors: Contemporary African American Academic Surgeons," *US National Library of Medicine*, https://www.nlm.nih.gov/exhibition/aframsurgeons/history.html, accessed August 10, 2016.

During the time of Washington, some white physicians would treat black patients, but only after all of their white patients were treated. Sometimes this took all day, often resulting in not getting to see them at all. Otherwise, black people would visit their local and unlicensed "root doctors." These were "the traditional healers and conjurers of the rural, black South." For further information, see: Wayland D. Hand, ed., *Popular Beliefs and Superstitions from North Carolina*, vols. 6 and 7 (1961, 1964) and Holly Matthews, "Doctors and Root Doctors: Patients Who Use Both," in James Kirkland and others, eds., *Herbal and Magical Medicine: Traditional Healing Today* (1992).

24. "Editorial," *The Southern Workman*, April 1921. Mrs. Bennet's first name is unknown.

25. John A. Kenney Sr. was medical director and chief surgeon at the Tuskegee Institute's John A. Andrew Memorial Hospital. His wife, Frieda Armstrong Kenney, graduated from Sargent School of Physical Education (Boston University) and taught at Tuskegee.

26. Elizabeth Brown, "The Career of Dr. John A. Kenney," *Campus Digest*, December 2, 1944.

27. "Dr. John A. Kenney Leaves Tuskegee." *Journal of the National Medical Association* 36.6 (1944): 199–200.

28. Mason's husband, Charles E., was at that time a member of Tuskegee University's Board of Trustees.

29. Rackham Holt, *George Washington Carver, An American Biography* (Garden City, NY: Doubleday and Co., 1943), 276. Robert R. Taylor was the first African

American to graduate from the Massachusetts Institute of Technology. He was also Booker T. Washington's chief architect, with the Tuskegee University Chapel seen as his greatest accomplishment. For further information see: Ellen Weiss, *Robert R. Taylor and Tuskegee: An African American Architect Designs for Booker T. Washington* (Montgomery, AL: New South Books, 2012).

30. The *Tuskegee Student* was the student newspaper for Tuskegee University.

31. "John A. Andrew Memorial Hospital," *Tuskegee Student*, Vol. 25, No. 5, 1913, 4.

32. Hildrus Poindexter was the first African American to receive both an MD at Harvard University in 1929 and a PhD in bacteriology at Columbia University in 1932. Poindexter later became the head of the Medical College at Howard University in 1934.

33. Hildrus A. Poindexter, *My World of Reality* (Detroit, MI: Balamp Publishing Co., 1973), 102.

34. For a brief overview of early black physicians, see: Miller, *John A. Kenney*, 63.

35. Louis W. Sullivan. "The Education of Black Health Professionals," *Phylon (1960–)*, Vol. 38, No. 2 (2nd Qtr., 1977), 183.

36. Howard University was founded in 1866 in response to the needs of post-Civil War freedmen that had moved to Washington, DC. Howard's first medical school opened in 1868 with eight students, seven black and one white. By 1881, the Freedman's Hospital had been established and constructed on the grounds of Howard University. For more information see: Herbert Morais. *The History of the Afro-American in Medicine*. Cornwells Heights, PA: The Publishing Agency, Inc., 1976. For information about Meharry Medical College, see: James Summerville, *Educating Black Doctors: A History of Meharry Medical College* (Tuscaloosa: University of Alabama Press, 2002).

37. Established specifically for the education and training of black physicians, Meharry Medical College, located in Nashville, Tennessee, was chartered in 1866 as part of the Central Tennessee College and its medical school opened in 1876 with less than a dozen students.

38. Abraham Flexner (1866–1959), a graduate of Johns Hopkins University, was an American educator whose report, published in 1910, helped to reform medical education in the United States. For further information, see: Thomas Neville Bonner, *Iconoclast: Abraham Flexner and a Life in Learning* (Baltimore: Johns Hopkins University Press, 2002). Note: Flexner was not a medical student and had no training in the field of medicine. Flexner spent two years at Johns Hopkins and earned a BA in Classics in 1886.

39. Morais, *Afro-American in Medicine*, 226–27.

40. By rural Southerners, the authors are speaking about both white and black people who lived in the South.

41. "Intertwined Destinies," *Montgomery Advertiser*, April 6, 1956.

42. These interns came to Tuskegee for training and experience even though they could not receive credit from any medical school.

43. The National Medical Association was founded in 1895 by black physicians as an alternative to the white-only American Medical Association. It was created by twelve black doctors at the Cotton States and International Exposition in Atlanta, Georgia. Robert F. Boyd was the first president and Daniel Hale Williams was the vice president. The organization's mission was to combat racism and segregation in

the medical field, both for medical professions and their patients. Quintard Taylor, "An Online Reference Guide to African American History," *BlackPast*, found on website www.blackpast.org/?q=aah/national-medical-association-1895. Accessed December 14, 2012.

44. Program of *The C.V. Roman Public Health Meeting* (Tuskegee, AL: Tuskegee Institute, April 1949), 4. The meeting was established as a memorial for C. V. Roman, one of the founders and first president of the John A. Andrew Clinical Society. Roman served as the first editor of the Journal of the National Medical Association. The journal was originally published at Tuskegee University, Alabama and was an outgrowth of the Negro National Medical Association with its first issue in January of 1909.

45. Contrarily, Dr. Kenney, in a speech before the NMA, noted, "we have banded ourselves together in the National Medical Association. We have no desire to be selfish or exclusive. There is not a phrase or word in our constitution or by-laws restricting membership to Negroes, nor will there ever be. Miller, *The Negro in Medicine, Updated*, 65.

46. This included, but was not limited to, education, public health, surgery, internal medicine, nursing, dentistry, and mental health.

47. Black physicians were also not eligible for membership in county and state medical societies.

48. Imes, *The Philosophies of Booker T. Washington*, 5–6.

49. "Intertwined Destinies," *Montgomery Advertiser*.

50. Many of these papers were published in the *Journal of the National Medical Association*.

51. *Birmingham News*, February 9, 1936.

52. Ibid.

53. "Board and lodging" were "furnished by Tuskegee Institute for $1.50 per day" and may have included payments to the private residences that provided overflow accommodations (Program, *The John A. Andrew Clinical Society*, 1927, 1). By 1954, the registration fee had increased to $10.00 (Program, *The John A. Andrew Clinical Society*, 1955, 50).

54. Drew was also examiner for the American Board of Surgery and a pioneer in the preservation of blood plasma.

55. The National Foundation for Infantile Paralysis was renamed The March of Dimes Birth Defects Foundation in 1976 (Maddock J. Baghdady, "Marching to a Different Mission," *Stanford Social Innovation Review*: 60–65 (Spring 2008). Retrieved December 11, 2012).

56. Editorial, *Montgomery Advertiser*.

57. Program, *John A. Andrew Clinical Society*, 1951, 32.

58. Ibid.

59. The films were not produced by the AMA, but were provided through a variety of companies, individuals, and organizations at no cost to the meeting.

60. Booker T. Washington, *Working With the Hands* (New York: Doubleday, Page & Company, 1904), 12.

61. Robert R. Moton, *Annals of the Academy of Political and Social Science*, 140: 257–263, n. 1928.

62. Sandra Crouse Quinn and Stephen B. Thomas "*The National Negro Health Week, 1915 to 1951: A Descriptive Account*," *Minority Health Today*, 2 (3), 2001, 44.

63. Ibid. Further reading: Monroe N. Work, *The Negro Year Book* (Tuskegee: Tuskegee, 1913–1943). These volumes are available at the Tuskegee University Archives.

64. Ibid., 44–49.

65. Roscoe C. Brown (1884–1962), served as the liaison between the USPHS and black communities. He was born in Washington, DC, on October 14, 1884, the son of John Robert and Blanche Maguire Brown. He was a graduate of M Street (later Dunbar) High School and received his degree from the College of Dentistry, Howard University, in 1906. He was one of the early dentists showing an interest in the social and public health aspects of dentistry. Dr. Brown played a major role in transferring the Office of Negro Health Work to the Special Programs Branch, Division of Health Education of the Public Health Service in 1950. He became the first chief of this new division and continued to give consultative services to black groups in their communities. He retired in 1954 at the age of 70.

66. From its inception in 1915, the Tuskegee oversight committee of the National Negro Health Week organized their activities with the support of other organizations such as the USPHS. "In 1921, the USPHS assumed publication of the NNHW Bulletin, and beginning in 1927 produced the Health Week Poster. Also in 1921, the first Annual NNHW conference, convened by the US Surgeon General, was held in Washington, DC. The purpose of the meeting, which included representatives of all cooperating agencies, was planning and evaluation of campaign activities." Quinn and Thomas, "The National Negro Health Week," 47–48. The takeover of the NNHW by the USPHS was a natural progression leading to increased and stable funding and dissemination of information to the public.

67. See, among others: W. D. Rasmussen, *Taking the University to the People: Seventy-five Years of Cooperative Extension* (Ames: Iowa State University, 1989); E. W. Crosby, "The Roots of Black Agricultural Extension Work," *Historian*, 39: 228–47 and *In The Beginning . . .*, George Washington Carver Center, USDA, 2009.

68. Thomas Monroe Campbell, *Movable School Goes to the Negro Farmer* (Tuskegee, AL: Tuskegee Institute Press, 1936), 79.

69. Even though there were similar such apparatus in Europe, this was innovative for the time in the South and amongst rural farmers, both black and white.

70. The National Grange had its beginnings in 1867 and "was aimed at assisting farmers in the South and West (their West is now our Mid-West)." Charles P. Gilliam, "A Short History of the Order of Patrons of Husbandry: The National Grange," http://www.oocities.org/cannongrange/cannon_nationalhistory.html, accessed July 28, 2016. The Farmers Alliance was "a fraternal organization of white farmers and other rural southerners, including teachers, ministers, and physicians, the Farmers' Alliance began in Texas in the mid-1870s and swept across the entire South during the late 1880s." Matthew Hild, "Farmer's Alliance," *New Georgia Encyclopedia*, http://www.georgiaencyclopedia.org/articles/history-archaeology/farmers-alliance, accessed July 28, 2016.

71. B. D. Mayberry, *Role of Tuskegee University in the Origin, Growth and Development of the Negro Cooperative Extension System, 1881–1990* (Montgomery, AL: Brown Printing Company, 1989), 28.

72. Ibid.

73. For more information, see: Marshall P. Wilder, *Address Delivered Before the Norfolk Agricultural Society, on the Occasion of its First Annual Exhibition, at Dedham*

(Boston: The Society, 1849); Charles G. Davis, "Historical Address" in Addresses Delivered at the Massachusetts Agricultural College, June 21st, 1887, on the 25th Anniversary of the Passage of the Morrill Land Grant Act (Amherst, Mass: J. E. Williams, 1887).

74. Land-grant funds under the Morrill Act consisted of monies acquired through the sale or use of 30,000 acres of federal land, either within or contiguous to its boundaries of each institution. These funds were to be specifically used to "teach such branches of learning as are related to agriculture and the mechanic arts, in such manner as the legislatures of the States may respectively prescribe, in order to promote the liberal and practical education of the industrial classes in the several pursuits and professions in life." Title 7, US Code, 307.

75. For more information, see: George B. Tindall, The Emergence of the New South, 1913–1945 (Baton Rouge: Louisiana State University Press, 1967).

76. Mayberry, Role, 37.

77. Ibid., 38.

78. James W. Smith, "The Contributions of Black Americans to Agricultural Extension and Research," found on website http://ageconsearch.umn.edu/bitstream/17424/1/ar840003.pdf. Accessed on December 8, 2015.

79. Title 7, US Code, 304.

80. Title 7, US Code, 343.

81. For more information, see: Roy Vernon Scott, The Reluctant Farmer: The Rise of Agricultural Extension to 1914 (Urbana: University of Illinois Press, 1971).

82. Greene was born in Gatesville, North Carolina and was an 1868 graduate of Hampton Institute, Virginia.

83. J. H. Palmer, "Farmer Greene," speech given at dedication of the Tuskegee University Extension Office Building, April 7, 1940, Tuskegee University Archives.

84. Mayberry, Role of Tuskegee, 38.

85. Ibid., 39.

86. Linda O. McMurray, George Washington Carver: Scientist and Symbol (Oxford, UK: Oxford University Press, 1981), 115.

87. Campbell, Movable School, 83.

88. Ibid.

89. Ibid., 39.

90. Alabama, Act To Establish Two Branch Agricultural Experiment Stations and Agricultural Schools for the Colored Race and to Make Appropriations Therefore (1897).

91. Ibid.

92. As the attached image shows, this "wagon" was similar in style to a modern Amish Surrey and not a wagon. Most Southerners considered a flatbed wagon with a single buckboard as a "wagon" with wheels of standard diameter.

93. Thomas Campbell, Movable School Goes to the Negro Farmer (Tuskegee, AL: Tuskegee Institute Press, 1936), 82.

94. Linda O. McMurry, George Washington Carver: Scientist and Symbol (Oxford, UK: Oxford University Press, 1981), 124.

95. Gwyn E. Jones and Chris Garforth, "The history, development, and future of agricultural extension," found on website http://www.fao.org/docrep/w5830e/w5830e03.htm. Accessed on December 15, 2015.

96. George Washington Carver to Booker T. Washington, November 16, 1904.

97. Mayberry, Role of Tuskegee, 55–56.

98. Campbell notes: the total cost of the Jesup Wagon and its equipment was $674.50. The items were two mules, $355.00; harness, $40.00; wagon, $190.50; cream separator, $75.00; two crates, $5.00; a revolving hand churn, $5.00; cultivator, $4.00. Campbell, *Movable School*, 93.

99. George Ruffum Bridgeforth (1873–1955) was born in Westmoreland, Alabama, on October 5, 1873. He was admitted to the Massachusetts Agricultural College in the fall of 1897. After graduation, Bridgeforth began his career in the Agricultural Department at Tuskegee in 1902 where he was appointed director of the department in 1904. After a decade at Tuskegee, he eventually taught in Topeka, Kansas, at the Industrial and Educational Institute. He would later move to Athens, Alabama, where he died on January 30, 1955.

100. White plantation owners felt the techniques promoted through the Jesup wagon's teachers could benefit them through increased yields and profits. For further information, see: Edmund Brunner and Hsin Pao Yang, *Rural America and the Extension Service* (New York: Bureau of Publications, Teachers College, Columbia University, 1949).

101. Mayberry, *Role*, 55–56.

102. Campbell, *Movable School*, 95.

103. Ibid., 97–98.

104. Ibid., 98–99.

105. The General Education Board (1902–1950) was a philanthropic organization that supported higher education and medical schools in the United States, aided rural white and black schools in the South, and helped to modernize farming practices in the South. For further information see: Raymond Blaine Fosdick, *Adventures in Giving: The Story of the General Education Board* (New York: Harper and Row, 1962).

106. The Slater Fund, formally known as The John F. Slater Fund for the Education of Freedmen, was created in the United States in 1882 for the encouragement of industrial education among Negroes in the South. For further information see: John E. Fisher, *The John F. Slater Fund: A Nineteenth Century Affirmative Action for Negro Education* (New York: University Press of America, 1986).

107. No doubt, Campbell was the right person for the job. He had served a variety of positions at Tuskegee, including driver, which familiarized him with the work of Washington, Carver, and Bridgeforth.

108. For more information, see: Nancy Woloch, *Women and the American Experience*, 5th ed. (New York: McGraw Hill, 2011) and Cheryl D. Hicks, *Talk with You like a Woman: African American Women, Justice, and Reform in New York, 1890–1925* (Chapel Hill: University of North Carolina Press, 2010).

109. Mayberry, *Role*, 99.

110. Campbell, *Movable School*, 108.

111. Ibid., 87. This is an example of the type of setting that Washington sought.

112. Booker T. Washington to David Franklin Houston, August 4, 1914.

113. Ibid.

114. Robert Zabawa, "Tuskegee Institute Movable School," Encyclopedia of Alabama, http://www.encyclopediaofalabama.org/article/h-1870#sthash.PinnBgF9 .dpuf. Accessed January 26, 2016.

115. Campbell, *Movable School*, 111.

116. Susan L. Smith, "Neither Victim Nor Villain," *Journal of Women's History*, 8 (1) (1996): 95.

117. Uva M. Hester, Weekly Report for Tuskegee Movable School, June 19, 1920.

118. For more information, see: Sharla Fett, *Working Cures: Healing, Health, and Power on Southern Slave Plantations* (Chapel Hill: University of North Carolina Press, 2002).

119. Probably similar, if not the same, to a "hoodoo man," a traditional African American folk healer that developed from a number of West African, Native American, and later on incorporating European, spiritual traditions, and beliefs. Carolyn Morrow Long, *Spiritual Merchants: Religion, Magic and Commerce* (Knoxville: University of Tennessee Press, 2001).

120. Campbell, *Movable School*, 116.

121. Campbell, *Movable School*, 122.

122. Mayberry, *Role*, 105.

123. Campbell, *Movable School*, 123.

124. Ibid., 152.

Chapter 2

Epigraph. *Robert Russa Moton of Hampton and Tuskegee*, ed. William Hardin Hughes and Frederick D. Patterson (Chapel Hill: University of North Carolina Press, 1956), 180.

1. *The Tuskegee Alumni Bulletin, 1920–1929*, 10.

2. "History," American Red Cross. Found on website http://www.redcross.org/about-us/who-we-are/history; accessed April 11, 2017.

3. McMurry, *George Washington Carver*, 203.

4. "Tuskegee Veterans Administration Hospital," Alabama Travel. Found on website http://www.alabama.travel/things-to-do/attractions/tuskegee_veterans_administration-hospital; accessed December 13, 2012.

5. For more information, see: Mary Kaplan, *The Tuskegee Veterans Hospital and Its Black Physicians: The Early Years* (Jefferson, NC: McFarland and Company, Inc., 2016) and Linda Kenney Miller, *Beacon on the Hill* (Dallas, TX: Harper House Publishers, 2008), 215–64.

6. James Jones, *Bad Blood: The Tuskegee Syphilis Experiment* (New York: Free Press, 1981), 64.

7. McMurray, *George Washington Carver*, 203–4.

8. Pete Daniel, "Black Power in the 1920s: The Case of the Tuskegee Veteran's Hospital," *Journal of Southern History* 36 (August 1970): 368–88.

9. "Tuskegee VA Medical Center Celebrates 85 Years of Service," *Central Alabama Veterans Health Care System*. Found on website http://www.centralalabama.va.gov/Press_Release.asp; accessed 13 December 2012.

10. McMurray, *George Washington Carver*, 203–4.

11. Daniel, "Black Power in the 1920s," 368–88.

12. "Tuskegee VA Medical Center Celebrates 85 Years of Service," press release, Central Alabama Veterans Health Care System (CAVHCS), accessed 13 December 2012.

13. Toussaint Tourgee Tildon (April 15, 1893–July 22, 1964), physician and psychiatrist, was born in Waxahachie, Texas, the son of John Wesley Tildon, a physician, and Margaret Hilburn. Tildon received a bachelor's degree from Lincoln University in Pennsylvania in 1912. He then studied pre-law at Harvard for one year

before entering medical school at Meharry Medical College in Nashville, Tennessee. He transferred to Harvard, earning an MD in 1923, specializing in psychiatry and neurology.

14. "A Good Work Goes Forward," *Birmingham News*, February 5, 1949.

15. Ibid.

16. "Sesquicentennial," *The Tuskegee News*, March 15, 1984.

17. The Macon County Hospital (1924–1980) continued as a "white hospital" until budgetary constraints in Macon County required its closure. Glenn Drummond, interviewed by the author, Tuskegee, Alabama, July 25, 2016.

18. Edith Powell and John F. Hume, *A Black Oasis: Tuskegee Institute's Fight Against Infantile Paralysis, 1941–1975* (Montgomery, AL: McQuick Printing, 2008), 1.

19. Forrest E. Ludden, *The History of Public Health in Alabama, 1941–1968* (Montgomery, AL: Alabama Department of Public Health, 1970), 16.

20. "County Health Departments," *Alabama Public Health*. Found on website http://www.adph.org/administration/Default.asp?id=505; accessed 25 February 2016.

21. Ludden, *Public Health in Alabama*, 35.

22. Rarely is Tuskegee's third president, Dr. Frederick D. Patterson, mentioned in the reports.

23. This section is not to be construed as a definitive exposé on eugenics or the works of Steggerda.

24. The concept of eugenics was propelled by the use of mathematical or analytical models in order to justify continued racial beliefs under the guise of "acceptable proof-outcomes." For more information see: Harold L. Aubrey, "African Americans and the Broader Legacy of Experience with the American Health Care Community: Parasites, Locusts, and Scavengers," ed. Ralph V. Katz and Rueben C. Warren, *The Search for the Legacy of the USPHS Syphilis Study at Tuskegee* (New York: Lexington Books, 2011), 110.

25. Davenport was born in Stamford, Connecticut. He attended Harvard University, earning a PhD in biology in 1892. In 1904, Davenport became director of Cold Spring Harbor Laboratory, where he founded the Eugenics Record Office in 1910.

26. Booker T. Washington to Charles Davenport, January 16, 1913.

27. Robert Norrell, *Up from History: The Life of Booker T. Washington* (New York: Belknap Press, 2011).

28. In The 1930s, Scientists Measured Black College Students To Define The "Negro Race," *BuzzFeed News*, http://www.buzzfeed.com/danvergano/tuskegee-student-measurements, accessed March 17, 2016.

29. Steggerda was born in Holland, Michigan. He received an AB from Hope College in 1922, and an AM and PhD from the Department of Zoology of the University of Illinois, in 1923 and 1928 respectively. His first position was an assistant professor of zoology at Smith College (1928–1930), but most of his career was spent as an investigator with the Carnegie Institution for Science at Cold Spring Harbor, New York (1930–1944). From then until his death of a heart attack on March 15, 1950, he was professor of anthropology at Hartford Seminary Foundation in Connecticut.

30. Anthropometry refers to the measurement of the human individual. It was an early tool of eugenics.

31. Lombardo, "Anthropometry, Race, and Eugenic Research," 232.

32. Charles Davenport to Robert R. Moton, April 3, 1933.

33. Cleveland "Cleve" Abbott was born in Yankton, South Dakota, in 1892. He received his bachelor's degree from South Dakota State University (SDSU) in Brookings, South Dakota, in 1916. He was an outstanding, multisport athlete in high school (16 varsity sports letters) and SDSU (14 varsity letters). He served in Europe in World War I as an officer in the 366th Infantry Regiment. Afterward he accepted a position as the eighth football coach at Tuskegee University. He held that position for thirty-two seasons, from 1923 until 1954.

34. Petty worked with Steggerda to coauthor articles on their work. See "An Anthropometric Study of Negro and White College Women."

35. In a letter to Robert R. Moton, dated February 10, 1932, Davenport mentioned that he would be at Tuskegee for "two or three days" because he was on the "way to the Yucatan." It is possible that Davenport stayed only those few days and afterward turned it over to Steggerda. Davenport would later write to Moton on April 3, 1933, that he was turning the work over to Morris Steggerda.

36. The finding aid from the Steggerda Collection at the National Museum of Health and Medicine, Silver Spring, Maryland, lists "Checking Sheets for Colton Valley, Harris Barrett and Rising Star" as some of the locations where measurements were taken. OHA 316 Steggerda Collection, Otis Historical Archives, *National Museum of Health and Medicine*, http://www.medicalmuseum.mil/assets/documents/collections/archives/2014/OHA%20316%20Steggerda%20Collection.pdf.

37. Items from collection titled "College Boys from Tuskegee Institute," Steggerda Collection, Box 31–00001 100, National Museum of Health and Medicine, Silver Spring, MD. Images found in same box.

38. "College Boys from Tuskegee Institute," Steggerda Collection, Box 31–00001 100, National Museum of Health and Medicine, Silver Spring, MD.

39. Moton to Steggerda, January 16, 1934.

40. This is confirmed by his work with the physical education department and Christine Petty, the women's coach, at Tuskegee University.

41. Lombardo, "Anthropometry, Race, and Eugenic Research," 230.

42. Faculty and Staff, *Tuskegee Institute Catalog*, 1935–1936.

43. Charles E. Rosenberg, *No Other Gods: On Science and American Social Thought* (Baltimore: Johns Hopkins University Press, 1997), 96. For more information on the rejection of eugenics by prominent biologists, see: T. H. Morgan to H. F. Osborn, June 14, 1920; William Bateson to C. B. Davenport, February 11, 1921, C. B. Davenport Papers. Jerry Bergman, in an article titled "A Brief History of the Eugenics Movement," *Investigator*, 2000 May, 77, states: "Although many prominent biologists in America and elsewhere remained committed to the basic eugenics program and the idea of a pure race until they died, many others quietly dropped their race ideas. Unfortunately, most scientists did not discuss the errors of their past much, even when the public tide turned strongly against the blatant racism of the movement as a whole. For most researchers, it became more and more apparent that many of the wholesale conclusions of the eugenicists were simply wrong. Once some of them were questioned, researchers began to question all of them. Soon the whole house of cards fell, and its fall was a near-total collapse."

44. Ibid., 89.

45. Lombardo, "Anthropometry, Race, and Eugenic Research," 301.

46. According to Harold L. Aubrey, the prevalent flaws in studies such as this

included "flaws in design, data collection, and interpretation." Aubrey, "African Americans," 114.

47. Max Seham. *Blacks and American Medical Care* (Minneapolis: University of Minnesota Press, 1973), 45. Morais notes: "From 1910 through 1947, these two schools graduated 3,439 students, 101 of whom were women." Morais, *Afro-American in Medicine*, 94.

48. Internships and residencies allowed medical students to specialize. Fields such as gynecology, pediatrics, obstetrics, neurology, etc., required specialized instruction and training before the doctor could obtain a license. This posed particular problems for the black physician. T. R. Payton, *Quest for Dignity: An Autobiography of a Negro Doctor* (Los Angeles: 1950).

49. Tuskegee Institute, *Annual Report of the President* (Tuskegee, AL: Tuskegee Institute Press, 1947), 9.

50. In order to placate black soldiers, in 1921 the Veterans Bureau and Tuskegee University agreed to construct a six hundred-bed hospital, including twenty-seven permanent structures, on 300 hundred acres of land leased by the university. Completed February 12, 1923, plans were initially made for an all-white staff, but were quickly changed due to the insistence of Tuskegee's second president, Robert R. Moton.

51. *New York Times* (article was taken from the Eugene Dibble Collection, Box 31, Folder 5, Tuskegee University Archives).

52. Powell and Hume, *A Black Oasis*, 101.

53. In 1914, General Hospital No. 2 was the first public hospital in the United States operated and staffed entirely by African Americans. Samuel Rodgers, "Kansas City General Hospital No. 2," *The Journal of the National Medical Association*, September 1, 525–44, 639.

54. John Franklin Hume (1915–2004) grew up in Brooklyn, New York. He received his undergraduate degree in physical education from City College of New York in 1936. He graduated from Howard University Medical School in 1940 and was accepted at Cleveland City Hospital as an intern, one of two African Americans, under the hospital's quota system. He took his residency in surgery at Freedman's Hospital and entered the Army in 1942. He completed his orthopedic training after the war, becoming the second black orthopedist to complete his boards and the second to be a member of the American Academy of Orthopaedic Surgeons (AAOS).

55. John Watson Chenault (1904–1965) was born in Sheridan, Wyoming. He received his Bachelor of Science in 1929, Bachelor of Medicine in 1930, and Doctor of Medicine in 1931, all from the University of Minnesota. Chenault was an orthopedic surgeon and served as director of orthopedics of the John A. Andrew Memorial Hospital. He served as director of the Infantile Paralysis Center from 1941–1942, 1946–1947, and 1952–1953.

56. Edith Powell and John Hume, *A Black Oasis: Tuskegee Institute's Fight Against Infantile Paralysis, 1941–1975* (Auburn, AL: Privately Published, 2009), 101.

57. Hume left for the VA hospital after the return of Dr. Chenault.

58. In the Veteran's Administration, the term "service" designates a department within the hospital.

59. Powell and Hume, *Black Oasis*, 102.

60. Ibid.

61. John A. Kenney, "Service of a Negro Hospital," *Southern Workman*, April 1921, 6–7.

62. For more information, see: Susan L. Smith, *Sick and Tired of Being Sick and Tired Black Women's Health Activism in America, 1890–1950* (Philadelphia: University of Pennsylvania Press, 1995).

63. Kenney, "Service," 9–10.

64. Kenney, "Second Annual Oration," 212.

65. Kenney, "Service," 9–10.

66. The Tuskegee Normal School for Nurses was established at the behest of Tuskegee University's first president, Booker T. Washington, in September 1892. The nursing school became a three-year program in 1908 and was registered in 1928 by the Alabama State Board of Nurse Examiners. In 1941, the school created a nurse practitioner program in midwifery and seven years later (1948) initiated the Bachelor of Science degree in nursing (BSN), the first in the state of Alabama and the first at a Historically Black College or University (HBCU). In the spring of 1953, fourteen African American students received their BSN. See Powell and Hume, *Black Oasis*, 7, for more information.

67. Lillian Harvey, interviewed by Edith Powell, October 13, 1986.

68. "Women of quality" meant a woman with a level of social status that permitted them to have someone else do things that they considered beneath them economically and socially. For more information: "Women's Roles in the 1950s." *American Decades*. Vol. 6. 2001. 278–80. Gale Group. 2005. July 16, 2008. http://find .galegroup.com.

69. This was one of many Jim Crow laws observed in several states from the 1880s to the 1960s. "Jim Crow Laws (Examples)," Martin Luther King, Jr., National Historic Site Interpretive Staff. 5 January 1998 http://www.nps.gove/malu/documents/jim_crow_laws.htm. For more information, see: Vanessa Northington Gamble, *Making a Place for Ourselves: The Black Hospital Movement, 1920–1945* (New York: Oxford University Press, 1995); Mitchell F. Rice and Woodrow Jones Jr., *Public Policy and the Black Hospital* (Westport, CT: Greenwood Press, 1994) and Thomas J. Ward Jr. *Black Physicians in the Jim Crow South* (Fayetteville: University of Arkansas Press, 2003).

70. In 1968, the National Foundation for Infantile Paralysis provided funds for a new building to house nursing students and faculty (now called Basil O'Connor Hall).

71. Powell and Hume, *Black Oasis*, 104.

72. Hines, Darlene Clark. *Black Women in White: Racial Conflict and Cooperation in the Nursing Profession, 1890–1950* (Bloomington: Indiana University Press, 1989). Also, *Tuskegee Institute Bulletin, 1949–50*, Tuskegee, 1950, 166.

73. The veterinary school is currently located adjacent to the hospital. This facilitated easy access to faculty and facilities by the nursing program.

74. The Infantile Paralysis wing of the hospital was dedicated in 1940 "for the treatment of victims of infantile paralysis and other crippling diseases." *Tuskegee Institute Bulletin, 1952–53*, Tuskegee, 1953, 168.

75. Lillian Harvey Collection, Box 42, Folder 4, Tuskegee University Archives. Pediatric polio victims were far from home and confined to beds that restricted them from play and extended visits from relatives. This caused a number of emotional and psychological problems for the children.

76. See, Naomi Rogers, "Race and the Politics of Polio: Warm Springs, Tuskegee, and the March of Dimes," *American Journal of Public Health*, May 2007, 97(5), 784–95. Rogers refers to: John W. Chenault, "Infantile Paralysis (Acute Anterior Poliomyelitis)," *Journal of the National Medical Association*, 33 (1941), 221.

77. John A. Kenney, "Service of a Negro Hospital," *Southern Workman*, April 1921.

78. Powell and Hume, *Black Oasis*, 29. In her book *Black Oasis*, Dr. Edith Powell notes that Eleanor Roosevelt and no doubt her husband, the president, were aware of the plight of African American children with polio as early as 1936. "On October 20, 1936, Mr. Walter White, Secretary to the NAACP, wrote to Mrs. Eleanor Roosevelt asking her advice in 'regard to admitting Negroes' to Warm Springs, Georgia . . . Mr. White informed Mrs. Roosevelt that the NAACP had refused to join in the President's Birthday Balls in 1934 because they could never get a satisfactory answer to their question concerning the status of Negroes who might apply for treatment." See for more information: Powell and Hume, *Black Oasis*, 32.

79. *The Infantile Paralysis Fight at Tuskegee* (New York: National Foundation for Infantile Paralysis, 1948), 5–8.

80. E. P. Davis to Eugene Dibble, May 11, 1949 (T.U. Archives, Dibble Collection, Box 32, Folder No. 1).

81. "Events 1901–1970," *Liberia*, Alabama Public Television. Found on website http://www.pbs.org/wgbh/globalconnections/liberia/timeline/time3.html; accessed 12 December 2012.

82. *President's Report*, 1947, 10.

Chapter 3

Epigraph 1. Chancellor Mark A. Nordenberg, *Defeat of an Enemy* (Pittsburgh: University of Pittsburgh Press, 2005), 15.

Epigraph 2. Shirley Graham and George D. Lipscomb, *Dr. George Washington Carver, Scientist* (New York: Simon & Schuster, Inc., 1972), 192.

1. David M. Oshinsky, *Polio: An American Story* (Oxford, UK: Oxford University Press, 2005).

2. Saul Benison quoted in: David Rose, *Images of America: March of Dimes* (Charleston, SC: Arcadia Publishing, 2003), 9. Saul Benison (1920–2006) was born in New York City. He graduated from Queens College in 1941, where he was the recipient of the K. S. Pinson Award in History. After serving as a historian for the War Production Board (1943–1945), he entered Columbia University's graduate history program in 1945. By the time he received his PhD in 1953, Benison had taught at the City College of New York, Sarah Lawrence College, and Long Island University. In 1968, he received the American Association for Medical History's William H. Welch Medal for distinguished achievement in medical historiography. Taken from: "In Memoriam," *American Historical Association Perspectives*, October 2007, 45:7.

3. Paintings and stone carvings show otherwise healthy adults and children with withered arms and legs. T. M. Daniel and F. C. Robbins, "A History of Poliomyelitis" *Polio* (Rochester, NY: University of Rochester Press, 1997), 5–22.

4. E. J. Sass, G. Gottfried, and A. Sore, *Polio's Legacy: An Oral History* (Washington, D.C: University Press of America, 1996).

5. Theo Lippman Jr., *The Squire of Warm Springs: F.D.R. in Georgia, 1924–1945* (Chicago: Playboy, 1977), 18.

6. For more information see: Jean Edward Smith, *FDR* (New York: Random House, 2008).

7. Meriwether Reserve was named after the Meriwether Inn (opened in the 1890s) on a thousand acres.

8. Nordenberg, *Defeat of an Enemy*, 14. Also, see: Oshinsky, *Polio: An American Story*. Oshinsky provides an in-depth discussion concerning Roosevelt's decision to go to Warm Springs, Georgia, and to create a nonprofit institution for the benefit of patients suffering from the effects of polio.

9. Lippman, *The Squire of Warm Springs*, 66.

10. Morgan was an accomplished insurance salesman in New York. He was associated with the Equitable Life Assurance Society as was his father before him. Equitable was known for decades as one of the largest life insurance companies in the nation. Morgan organized the Birthday Ball program from 1934 to 1945, every year of its existence. He also served as treasurer of the Georgia Warm Springs Foundation and was a cofounder of the National Foundation for Infantile Paralysis with F. D. R. and Basil O'Connor.

11. David Oshinsky, *Polio: An American Story* (Oxford, UK: Oxford University Press, 2005), 47.

12. The stock market crash of 1929 was actually an event that continued over a four-year period, which included the Great Depression of 1932–1933.

13. Oshinsky, *Polio: An American Story*, 47.

14. Carl Robert Byoir (1886 –1957), was born to Jewish immigrant parents from Poland, but raised in Des Moines, Iowa. Byoir started his career in public relations at 14 as a reporter for *The Des Moines Register*. At the age of 17, he became the editor of the *Waterloo Times-Tribune*. He worked his way through the University of Iowa while he was the circulation manager for Hearst Magazine's publications. In 1930, he created one of the largest public-relations firms in the world.

15. Apparently, there has been some discrepancy regarding the name of this original celebration. Some authors contend that it was called "the Committee for the Celebration for the President's Birthday." The F. D. R. Library and Museum call it the "National Committee for Birthday Balls."

16. Ibid., 50.

17. Ibid., 53.

18. Jane S. Smith, *Patenting the Sun: Polio and the Salk Vaccine, the Dramatic Story Behind One of the Greatest Achievements of Modern Science* (New York: William Morrow and Company, Inc., 1990), 70–73.

19. Rose, *March of Dimes: Images of America*, 9.

20. Lippman, *The Squire of Warm Springs*, 208.

21. Oshinsky, *Polio: An American Story*, 53.

22. Born in New York, Cantor appeared in the "Ziegfeld Follies" and was famous for his eye-rolling song-and-dance routines. He wrote and performed several songs including: "Ma! He's Makin' Eyes at Me," and "Merrily We Roll Along," the *Merrie Melodies* Warner Bros. cartoon theme. He was best known for his variety radio show and then particularly as a philanthropist and humanitarian.

23. Gregory Koseluk, *Eddie Cantor: A Life in Show Business* (Jefferson, NC: McFarland & Company, 1995).

24. Helen Hayes, *My Life in Three Acts* (San Diego: Harcourt Brace Jovanovich, 1990).

25. Rose, Images of America, 49.

26. The staff became more focused on treatment and rehabilitation. Early in the 1940s, techniques developed by medical professionals such as Dr. Howard A. Rusk and nurse Sister Kenny, led to new methods of treatment and rehabilitation. The doctors and nurses at Warm Springs utilized these techniques, expanding them to fit their own needs. For further information, see: John R. Paul, *A History of Poliomyelitis* (New Haven: Yale University Press, 1971).

27. Rose, *Images of America*, 9.

28. Ibid.

29. Bettyann O'Connor Culver had contracted the disease in July 1950. Ibid., 40.

30. Ibid., 2.

31. As previously noted, Basil O'Connor served as chairman of the Tuskegee Institute Board of Trustees from 1946 to 1968.

32. *Four Eulogies* (White Plains, NY: The National Foundation-March of Dimes, 1972).

33. Ibid.

34. Smith, *Patenting the Sun*, 86.

35. For more, see: B. D. Mayberry, *The History of the Carver Research Foundation of Tuskegee University* (Tuskegee, AL: Tuskegee University Press, 2003).

36. Peter Duncan Burchard, *George Washington Carver: For His Time and Ours* (Diamond, Missouri: United States Department of the Interior Printing, 2005), 1.

37. Holt, *George Washington Carver*, 298. Note: A "rubber" is similar to an athletic trainer today. Carver worked to alleviate cramps, bruises, and sore muscles that plagued athletes at that time.

38. Eugene H. Dibble Jr., M.D. (1893–1968) served in the army during both World Wars and was commissioned colonel in the Army Medical Corps from 1944–1946. He was manager of the United States Veterans Administration Hospital at Tuskegee from 1936–1946; medical director of the John A. Andrew Memorial Hospital from 1946–1965; and served as a member of the Board of Trustees at Meharry Medical College in Nashville, Tennessee. Dr. Dibble also served as Secretary of the John A. Andrew Clinical Society from 1924–1926 and 1946–1965.

39. George Washington Carver to Eugene Dibble, December 3, 1934.

40. Ibid.

41. George Washington Carver to Miss Chisholm, December 29, 1934.

42. George Washington Carver to Mrs. Mays, March 19, 1935.

43. George Washington Carver to M. L. Ross, April 19, 1935.

44. T. M. Davenport, "Peanut Oil Helps Victims of Paralysis," Associated Press, December 31, 1933.

45. Powell, *A Black Oasis*, 16.

46. Franklin Delano Roosevelt to George Washington Carver, April 7, 1939. This occurred during Roosevelt's visit to Tuskegee University and the GWCRF in March 1939.

47. For more information on this, see: C. Lewis Wrenshall, "The American Peanut Industry," *Economic Botany*, III (April–June 1949), 168; Robin Bird to William R. Carroll, July 6, 1961; C. H. Fisher to Carroll, October 20, 1961. Also, see: William R. Carroll and Merle E. Muhrer, "The Scientific Contributions of George Wash-

ington Carver" (unpublished report for National Park Service, 1962). All of these can be found in the Papers of George Washington Carver, Tuskegee University Archives, Tuskegee, Alabama.

48. Elizabeth Kenny (1880–1952) was an Australian nurse whose controversial approach to the treatment of poliomyelitis included heat and vigorous exercising of muscles affected by polio. Her principles of muscle rehabilitation were later adopted by the NFIP and became the foundation of physical therapy, or physiotherapy. John F Pohl, MD, with Elizabeth Kenny, *The Kenny Concept of Infantile Paralysis, and Its Treatment* (St. Paul, MN: Bruce Publishing Co., 1943).

49. Prescription, J. F. Fargason, MD, to George Washington Carver, May 27, 1935.

50. George Washington Carver to L. C. Fischer, June 24, 1935.

51. L. C. Fischer to George Washington Carver, July 7, 1935.

52. Ethel Edwards, *Carver of Tuskegee* (Tuskegee, Alabama: Privately Published, 1971), 202.

53. *Annual Report of the George Washington Carver Foundation and a Resume of the Period, 1940–1947* (Tuskegee, AL: Tuskegee Institute, 1948), 1.

54. Austin Wingate Curtis Jr. (1911–2004) was assistant to Dr. George Washington Carver from 1935–1943 and director of the George Washington Carver Foundation, 1943–1944.

55. Edwards, *Carver of Tuskegee*, 198.

56. B. D. Mayberry, *The History of the Carver Research Foundation of Tuskegee University 1940–1990* (Tuskegee, AL: Tuskegee University Press, 1990), ix.

57. Ibid.

58. For further information on the financing of the facility, see: Ibid., 28–29.

59. Carver Research Foundation.

60. Mayberry, *The History of the Carver Research Foundation*, ix. Although Mayberry (and many other writers) often used the honorific "Dr." when referring to George Washington Carver, Carver never actually earned a doctorate.

Chapter 4

Epigraph. Laurie Garrett, *Betrayal of Trust: The Collapse of Global Public Health* (New York: Hyperion, 2011), 139.

1. An infectious agent may include a virus, bacteria, or fungus. Mark Peakman and Diego Vergani, *Basic and Clinical Immunology, 2nd Edition* (London: Churchill Livingstone, 2009).

2. Efficacy is defined as how well the vaccines work.

3. Depending on the situation, such as in the case of the Ebola vaccine, the "FDA is working to help expedite the development and availability of medical products—such as treatments, vaccines, diagnostic tests, and personal protective equipment—with the potential to help bring the Ebola epidemic in West Africa under control as quickly as possible." This can measurably shorten the amount of time for the availability of a vaccine. "Protecting and Promoting Your Health," *US Food and Drug Administration*, http://www.fda.gov/EmergencyPreparedness/Counterterrorism/MedicalCountermeasures/ucm410308.htm. Accessed on March 7, 2016.

4. Media plates are containers with some recipe of biochemicals (or laboratory media) that are known to support or kill the growth of the infectious agent.

5. Host means the body. Morag C. Timbury, *Notes on Medical Virology* (London: Churchill Livingstone, 1994), 7.

6. Smith, *Patenting the Sun*, 96.

7. Antibody titer is a laboratory test that measures the concentration of the number or level of antibodies in a blood sample. Timbury, *Notes on Medical Virology*, 28–29.

8. Martinus Willem Beijernick was a Dutch microbiologist and botanist who started the Delft School of Microbiology.

9. Wendell Meredith Stanley was an American biochemist, virologist and Nobel Laureate.

10. Alexis Carrel was a French surgeon, biologist, and Nobel Laureate, known as the "father of *in vitro* tissue culture (which is the process of growing cells outside of the body)."

11. Ian R. Tizard, *Immunology: An Introduction* (Philadelphia: Saunders College Publishing, 1995), 5–6.

12. Smith, *Patenting the Sun*, 97.

13. Albert Bruce Sabin (1906–1993) was a Polish American medical researcher.

14. "By the mid-1930s several animal viruses had been cultured in laboratory flasks, as well as in the developing of chicken embryos of fertile eggs." Ibid., 125.

15. John Franklin Enders, called "The Father of Modern Vaccines," was an American biomedical scientist and Nobel laureate.

16. Nutrients are constituents of food necessary for normal physiologic function. Michael Madigan and John Martinko, eds., *Brock Biology of Microorganisms* (11th ed.) (Cranbury, NJ: Prentice Hall, 2005).

17. "Nobel Lectures," *Physiology or Medicine 1942–1962* (Amsterdam, Elsevier Publishing Company, 1964).

18. *A Paralyzing Fear: The Story of Polio in America*, DVD, directed by Nina Gilden Seavey (1998; Burbank, CA: Public Broadcasting System (PBS), 1998).

19. Smith, *Patenting the Sun*, 109.

20. "This typing or 'fingerprinting' of virus required a huge investigation by research teams [from four laboratories] . . . Testing 100 strains of virus collected from over the world, they spent three years' time, $1,370,000 in March of Dimes funds, and employed 30,000 monkeys." *A Paralyzing Fear*, PBS.

21. Oshinsky, *Polio: An American Story*, 118.

22. Alton Blakeslee, *Polio Can Be Conquered* (Washington: Public Affairs Committee, Incorporated, 1949), 19–20. "It had been previously thought that the virus entered the body through the nose and went straight to the nervous tissue, bypassing the blood stream. If that was the case, there would be no way a vaccine could be made. Antibodies are detected in the blood, so if the virus did not go into the blood stream, no antibodies would be produced or triggered by the cells in the blood stream. This new discovery meant that the virus entered the mouth carried by fecal contamination of the hands or water, then into the blood stream." Also, see: *A Paralyzing Fear*, PBS.

23. "Nobel Lectures," Physiology or Medicine 1942–1962.

24. The electron microscope was coinvented by two Germans, Max Knoll and Ernst Ruska, in 1931. Ernst Ruska was awarded half of the Nobel Prize for Physics in 1986 for his invention.

25. It was determined that babies up to six months old were protected by antibodies from the mother that passed through the placenta and stayed in the baby's bloodstream for up to six months. At that time the baby's immune system could start building its own antibodies when exposed to a virus.

26. Smith, *Patenting the Sun*, 100.

27. Ibid., 101.

28. Jonas Edward Salk was born in New York City to parents who were Jewish Russian immigrants.

29. Francis was an American physician, virologist, and epidemiologist who became the first person to isolate influenza virus in America. In 1940, while working at Mount Sinai Hospital, he showed that there are other strains of influenza and took part in the development of influenza vaccines. Francis left Mount Sinai Hospital at New York University (NYU) and, in 1942, joined the University of Michigan as director of the School of Public Health.

30. For more information, see: John Bankston, *Jonas Salk and the Polio Vaccine* (Bear, Delaware: Mitchell Lane Publishers, 2002), 30–32.

31. Oshinsky, *Polio: An American Story*, 110.

32. Bodian was at Johns Hopkins at this time.

33. Francis was at University of Michigan.

34. Sabin was at University of Cincinnati.

35. Oshinsky, *Polio: An American Story*, 110.

36. Teri Shors, *Understanding Viruses* (Burlington, MA: Jones and Bartlett Publishers, 2008).

37. Dave Preston to Charles Bynum, November 17, 1954, Archives, March of Dimes, White Plains, NY.

38. Ibid.

39. *The National Foundation for Infantile Paralysis News*, Sunday, January 16, 1955.

40. Harry M. Weaver (1908–1977) was the director of research for the NFIP from 1946 to 1953. His two major accomplishments during that time were to create a method of calculating indirect costs in the research grants program of the NFIP and to orchestrate the efforts in vaccine research that ultimately led to the development of the Salk polio vaccine. He was responsible for inviting Jonas Salk to an NFIP meeting to discuss the poliovirus typing project that led to Salk's association with the NFIP. Weaver was born in Lancaster, Ohio, on March 20, 1908 and received his AB, MSc, and PhD degrees from Ohio State University. He resigned from the NFIP in 1953, leaving in controversy over the planning of the Salk vaccine field trial. David Oshinsky, in *Polio: An American Story*, characterizes Weaver on pp. 112–15 *et seq* very nicely.

41. Smith, *Patenting the Sun*, 111.

42. Ibid., 172.

43. "Poliomyelitis Vaccine Types 1, 2, and 3," *Recommendations of Vaccine Advisory Committee*, National Foundation for Infantile Paralysis, April 25, 1954.

44. Established in 1953, this committee was responsible for planning the largest medical experiment ever attempted, the Salk vaccine field trials. Members included health experts from the federal government and academia, including those from the private sector. Oshinsky, *Polio: An American Story*, 171–73.

45. The items reproduced from this list are not sequentially numbered (they

were items 3, 4, 7, 8, 15, 17, and 18). Only those points germane to the text were included, and we changed the numbers to bullets to avoid the nonsequential list.

46. *Recommendations of Vaccine Advisory Committee*, 1–10.

47. Inactivated (killed) viruses are those that are heated and treated by radiation or chemicals until they are no longer able to reproduce within the living cell.

48. Live virus vaccines are made from viruses bred to be particularly weak. Breeding or attenuation takes place in the laboratory as the disease is passed from culture to culture.

49. Smith, *Patenting the Sun*, 199–201.

50. Ibid., 242.

51. Hart Van Riper was medical director of what is now the NFIP when it underwrote the drive to wipe out infantile paralysis, or poliomyelitis. Hart Van Riper was born in Kirkwood, Illinois. He graduated in 1926 from the University of Pennsylvania, where he received his medical degree in 1930. He practiced pediatrics and was medical director of an insurance company in Madison, Wisconsin, through the 1930s. He worked in the Children's Bureau of the Labor Department in Washington before joining the National Foundation for Infantile Paralysis in New York in 1945. He was its medical director until 1956. He then was medical director and vice president for medical affairs of Geigy Pharmaceuticals in Ardsley, N.Y., until 1970.

52. Smith, *Patenting the Sun*, 201–2.

53. A placebo is a substance containing no medication and prescribed or given to reinforce a patient's expectation to get well.

54. Following the conclusion of the vaccine inoculations, every case of polio (paralytic, nonparalytic, suspect, or doubtful) was to be immediately reported for any child in the spring of 1954 whether they had been inoculated or not. This was the responsibility of the community medical providers. Thomas Francis, et al., *Evaluation of the 1954 Field Trial of Poliomyelitis Vaccine: Final Report* (Ann Arbor, MI: Edwards Brothers, Inc., 1957), 77.

55. In the world of big drug companies, there is usually a minimum of ten years of research before a drug can be brought to the market, and during that time period, the company has to pay salaries, buy supplies, provide space, and deal with the voluminous amount of administrative work required in getting approval from the FDA. Only after the new drug is patented and put into the stores can the company begin to recoup the dollars that have been paid out during the research time when no money was coming in. This accounts for the two to three or more hundred percent mark-up passed on to the public for the cost of the new drug. For further information, see: A. S. Pina, A. Hussain, A. C. Roque, "An historical overview of drug discovery," *Methods of Molecular Biology*, 2009;572:3–12.

56. Thomas Francis Jr. was a physician, virologist, and epidemiologist. He was the first person to isolate influenza virus in America. In 1940, he showed that there are other strains of influenza and took part in the development of influenza vaccines.

57. Francis, *Evaluation of the 1954 Field Trial*, 28–29.

58. Smith, *Patenting the Sun*, 232.

59. Ibid.

60. Francis, *Final Report*, 35–36.

61. Ibid., 36.

62. Naomi Rogers. "Public Health Then and Now: Race and the Politics of

Polio: Warm Springs, Tuskegee, and the March of Dimes" *American Journal of Public Health*, May, 2007, Vol. 97, No. 5, 795.

63. Ibid. 784–95.

64. Although it is unclear exactly who sponsored this event, it was a fund-raiser as part of the NFIP's efforts to raise money for a polio vaccine as evidenced by the dimes on hats and cards.

65. Ibid.

66. Rose, *Images of America*, 9.

67. Charles Hudson Bynum (1905–1996), was born in Kinston, North Carolina. Prior to joining the March of Dimes, he was a high school biology teacher; dean of Texas College in Tyler, Texas; and assistant to President Frederick Patterson of Tuskegee Institute in Tuskegee, Alabama.

68. For more information, see: David W. Rose, *Friends and Partners: The Legacy of Franklin D. Roosevelt and Basil O'Connor in the History of Polio* (Boston: Academic Press, 2016).

69. Stephen E. Mawdsley, "Dancing on Eggs': Charles H. Bynum, Racial Politics, and the National Foundation for Infantile Paralysis, 1938–1954," *Bulletin of the History of Medicine*, 84, 2 (Summer 2010): 217.

70. A native of Guadaloupe, French West Indies, Paul Bertau Cornely (1906–2002) received his MD in 1931 at the University of Michigan Medical School. In 1934, he received his PhD in Public Health at Michigan. He taught at the Howard School of Medicine from 1934 until his retirement in 1973.

71. The first poster featured Rita Reed, from Blue Island, Illinois. Source: March of Dimes Archives, White Plains, NY.

72. See appendix 1 for a list of all African American Polio Poster Children (1947–1960).

73. Mawdsley, " 'Dancing on Eggs,' " 241.

74. Rogers, "Race and the Politics of Polio," 785.

75. Ibid.

76. For more detailed information, see appendix 2.

77. This facility was located at the University of Michigan on request of the NFIP. The NFIP felt that this would provide the study with an objective and unbiased evaluation of the data.

78. Alton L. Blakeslee, *Polio and the Salk Vaccine: What You Should Know About It* (New York: Gossett and Dunlap, 1956), 32–37.

79. John Troan, "How 'fooling around with polio thing' led to a medical miracle," *Pittsburgh Tribune-Review*, April 3, 2005.

Chapter 5

Epigraph. Dave Preston to Charles Bynum, November 17, 1954.

1. The first successful result of an in vitro culture was by Hanning (1904) who obtained transplantable seedings and grew (under aseptic conditions) some relatively mature embryos of *Raphanus*, *R. landra*, *R. sativus*, and *cochleasia danica (Brassicacesae)* on Tollens medium with sugars, amino acids, and plants extracts. Mehetre, S. S; Aher, A. R. (2004). "Embryo rescue: A tool to overcome incompatible interspecific hybridization in *Gossypium* Linn, A review," *Indian Journal of Biotechnology* 3: 29–36.

2. There were 27 grantee laboratories working for the NFIP; some elected to use monkey cells in lieu of the HeLa cells. Dave Preston to Charlie Bynum, November 17, 1954, Archives, March of Dimes, White Plains, NY.

3. Rebecca Skloot, *The Immortal Life of Henrietta Lacks* (New York: Crown Publishing Group, a Division of Random House, 2010).

4. George Otto Gey (July 6, 1899–November 8, 1970) and his wife, Margaret K. (1900–1989), started the Tissue Culture Laboratory at Johns Hopkins University in the 1950s.

5. Also known as stage one malignant epidermoid carcinoma.

6. J. Katz, *The Silent World of Doctor and Patient* (Baltimore: Johns Hopkins University Press, 2002), 2.

7. Ibid.

8. Cobbs v. Grant (8 Cal. 3d 229) 1972, *Law and Bioethics*, http://www .lawandbioethics.com/demo/Main/LegalResources/C5/Cobbs.htm, accessed May 18, 2014.

9. Jessica De Bord, "Informed Consent," Ethics in Medicine, University of Washington School of Medicine, 2014, https://depts.washington.edu/bioethx/topics/ consent.html, accessed June 12, 2014.

10. Elisa Eiseman and Susanne B. Haga, *Handbook of Human Tissue Sources: A National Resource of Human Tissue Samples* (Santa Monica, CA: Rand Corporation, 1999), xvii.

11. Skloot, *The Immortal Life*, 316.

12. Ibid., 17.

13. Ibid., 33.

14. The George Washington Carver Foundation began in 1943, upon Carver's death, with his life's savings as the impetus. The foundation was built upon the idea of giving black students a venue to work within without the stigma of racism and segregation. The building, completed in 1952, gave scientists a viable area to work with their experiments.

15. Basil O'Connor, *Address to Commemorate the Tuskegee Infantile Paralysis Center's Tenth Anniversary*, November, 1950.

16. *Final Report*, 115.

17. Ibid., 116.

18. Russell W. Brown, William F. Scherer, et al., "Report: The Ubiquitous HeLa Cell: Historic Account of the Mass Production and Distribution of HeLa Cells and Prototype Animal Cell Repository at Tuskegee Institute," Grant No. 1–753, March of Dimes/Birth Defects Foundation, March 1, 1981, 5.

19. Okatie Farms in Pritchardville, South Carolina, was established by the NFIP and Basil O'Connor to provide a "rest station" or clearinghouse for primates for the virus typing program. Since supply and disease were the main concerns of the scientists, the monkeys would be bought by the foundation and shipped from India or other points of origin, to Okatie Farms to rest and be checked for diseases. Then they would be shipped out to laboratories around the country. Smith, *Patenting the Sun*, 121.

20. MOD, Box CRBS4, File CRBS (CVRE) April 19, Tuskegee Institute, 1953.

21. There were several drafts/revisions of this paper leading up to the final version that was actually published. The final version did not include much of the information given in the preliminary versions. This version, along with several others, can be found in the "Papers of Russell Brown," Tuskegee University Archives.

"The Ubiquitous HeLa Cell: Historic Account of the Mass Production and Distribution of HeLa Cells at Tuskegee Institute, 1953–1955," subsequent drafts/revisions also bear the same title. There are no surviving members of the team working with Drs. Brown and Henderson (both of whom are deceased), therefore prompting the authors to rely upon the materials at the archives and at the March of Dimes archives.

22. The inconsistencies primarily revolve around Jimmy Henderson's participation with the project. Further documentation and correspondence reveal that Henderson's participation was limited at best. Henderson did not spend more than a few weeks for training, unlike Brown whose was extensive. Henderson's work was primarily with plant cells, not human.

23. In 1926 Russell W. Brown (1905–1985) received a BS degree at Howard University, where he majored in liberal arts, which included a wide selection of undergraduate courses. During 1929–1930, as a graduate student at the University of Chicago, he continued the liberal arts tradition by pursuing a variety of biomedical science courses, such as bacteriology, histology, embryology, physiology, and laboratory diagnostic methods. Subsequently, Brown received his MS in 1932 and PhD in 1936, with a major in physiological bacteriology and minor in biochemistry at Iowa State University.

24. James H. M. Henderson (1925–2009) received his BS degree from Howard University in 1939, MPh in 1940, and PhD in 1943 from the University of Wisconsin, with a major in plant biochemistry. He came to Tuskegee Institute in 1945 from the University of Chicago Toxicity Laboratory, National Defense Research Committee, Chemical Warfare Service.

25. March of Dimes Archives.

26. *Minutes of the Annual Meeting*, Board of Directors, George Washington Carver Foundation, February 10, 1953.

27. Roy C. Newton was an American food scientist who was involved in research and development of antioxidants in food and meat products during the twentieth century. He also was a founding member of the Institute of Food Technologists (IFT) in 1939.

28. *Minutes of the Annual Meeting*, GWCF, February 10, 1953.

29. Each summer, the Tissue Culture Association met at Cooperstown, New York, in order to teach basic methods of cellular cultivation. *An Introduction to Cell and Tissue Culture, By the Staff of the Tissue Culture Course, Cooperstown, New York, 1949–1953* (Minneapolis, MN: Burgess Publishing Co., 1955).

30. Scherer and Syverton to the NFIP, May 2, 1953. March of Dimes Archives.

31. Ibid.

32. In a proposal to the March of Dimes/Birth Defects Foundation titled *Historic Documentation of HeLa Cell Mass Production*, Tuskegee Institute, February 1981, Henderson was not originally included as one of the authors of the published report. The proposal noted: "It will be necessary to examine all of this material, extract the essential information and prepare a manuscript acceptable for a refereed publication. It is proposed that this be done by Dr. Russell W. Brown, the original project director, in consultation with Dr. William F. Scherer and with the assistance of Dr. Linda P. Washington, cell biologist, of the Tuskegee faculty." Furthermore, in the grant budget proposal, Henderson was not included in any of the line items. March of Dimes Grant no. 1–753. March of Dimes Archives.

33. Russell W. Brown and James H. M. Henderson, unpublished draft: "The

Ubiquitous HeLa Cell: Historic Account of the Mass Production and Distribution of HeLa Cells at Tuskegee Institute, 1953–1955," 6. Tuskegee University Archives. From here on, this document will be referred to as "unpublished draft."

34. Russell W. Brown had relinquished his position as director of the CRF so as to work specifically on the HeLa project. Ibid., 4.

35. Ibid., 6.

36. Ibid., 7.

37. Scherer's cell culture originated with Dr. Gey, in 1951 at Johns Hopkins Hospital.

38. Brown and Henderson, Unpublished Draft, 7–10.

39. The HeLa project was in fact responsible for several innovations in laboratory supplies such as rubber-lined screw-capped tubes and bottles, which led to large-quantity special deliveries.

40. Brown and Henderson, Unpublished Draft, 8.

41. See appendix 3 for a complete listing of laboratory staff at Tuskegee University during the production of strain HeLa for the Salk vaccine field trials.

42. Colony counts use petri dishes containing media that will support bacteria growth. They are left in the area to be tested with the top off. Air settles onto the media and bacteria, if present, will grow on the media. The dish is covered and incubated at 37 degrees centigrade (98.6° F). From a grid located on the petri dish, bacteria colonies are counted and the resultant figure determines the level of contamination. Air quality is then adjusted accordingly.

43. Brown and Henderson, Unpublished Draft, 9. There is no description of the facility outside of that given in the unpublished draft of Brown and Henderson.

44. According to the brief sketch in *American Journal of Digestive Diseases*, May 1953, Dr. Kumm was born in Wiesbaden, Germany. He came to the United States via Britain and became an American citizen in 1945. He had spent twenty-three years on the staff of the Rockefeller Foundation for Medical Research before joining the NFIP in July 1951. In May 1953, Dr. Kumm replaced Dr. Harry M. Weaver as director of polio research at NFIP.

45. Scherer to Kumm, November 6, 1953, March of Dimes Archives.

46. Microbiological Associates, which later became a part of biotech giants Invitrogen and BioWhittaker, created the first industrial for-profit cell distribution center.

47. Scherer to Kumm, January 27, 1954. March of Dimes Archives.

48. Kumm to Scherer, February 3, 1954. March of Dimes Archives.

49. Multiple authors, October to December 1953. March of Dimes Archives.

50. An autoclave is used in the medical field to sterilize equipment and media by increased temperature and pressure.

51. Scherer to Kumm, February 15, 1953. March of Dimes Archives.

52. Syverton to Francis, March 26, 1954. March of Dimes Archives.

53. See appendix 4 for a list of the grantee laboratories involved in the field trials testing of the vaccine evaluation program.

54. Brown and Henderson, Unpublished Draft, 16.

55. Brown and Henderson, Unpublished Draft, 9.

56. The BD Cornwall Disposable Syringe system offers a user-friendly design for accurate, efficient, comfortable fluid transfer. It is a manual, sterile device that has a two-way valve that attaches to both the syringe and the solution to be drawn

into the syringe. Releasing the grips fills the syringe with solution; compressing the grip expels the syringe contents.

57. Brown and Henderson, Unpublished Draft, 14.

58. Ibid.

59. Brown further wrote: "We made the first shipment to Scherer and Syverton on 21 September 1953 by parcel post, special handling, and it was received in Minneapolis on 25 September." Ibid., 15. This, too, proved unreliable.

60. Ibid., 13.

61. Brown noted: "From our first experimental shipments to Dr. Scherer at Minneapolis we learned that the results were most satisfactory when the tube and bottle monolayers were given fresh medium one day before shipment, the medium removed just before packaging, and the shipping time did not exceed two days." Ibid., 12.

62. Hart E. Van Riper to Basil O'Connor, October 22, 1953, March of Dimes Archives.

63. Mária Telkes (1900–1995) was a Hungarian-American scientist and inventor who worked on solar energy technologies. Telkes was considered one of the founders of solar thermal storage systems. She moved to Texas in the 1970s and consulted with a variety of start-up solar companies, including Northrup Solar, which subsequently became ARCO Solar and eventually BP Solar.

64. J. N. Ashworth graduated from Brown University in 1942 and earned his PhD in chemistry from the University of Wisconsin in 1948. He became assistant director of the Red Cross Blood Program on December 1, 1952. Biographical information on J. N. Ashworth compiled by Office of Public Relations, American National Red Cross, National Archives at College Park, Maryland.

65. T. E. Boyd to Maria Telkes, October 1, 1953, March of Dimes Archives.

66. For more information, see correspondence: Renato Contini to Theodore E. Boyd, September 24, 1053. T. E. Boyd to Renato Contini, October 2, 1953, March of Dimes Archives.

67. John F. Enders to T. E. Boyd, October 13, 1954, March of Dimes Archives.

68. "Sample of letter sent to all recipient laboratories," Russell W. Brown, January 27, 1955, March of Dimes Archives. Questionnaires, with attached letter for R. W. Brown, were designed with carbon copies so that all parties could have access to the information that they provided.

69. R. W. Brown to T. E. Boyd, October 21, 1954, March of Dimes Archives.

70. Ibid.

71. Brown and Henderson, Unpublished Draft, 16. For more information see footnote number 382.

72. Ibid., 16.

Chapter 6

Epigraph. Imes, *The Philosophies of Booker T. Washington*, 11.

1. See more at: http://www.polioeradication.org/Infectedcountries.aspx#sthash .SSASd2Gk.dpuf.

2. *Tuskegee Institute Annual Report of the President, 1955–1956*, 32.

3. "Crippling statistics: Fight against militants leads to polio spike," *International Herald Tribune*, Jan. 15, 2011.

4. Hilary Koprowski (1916–2013) was a Polish and American virologist and immunologist.

5. "Hilary Koprowski, Who Developed First Live-Virus Polio Vaccine, Dies at 96," *New York Times*, April 20, 2013.

6. Although the ethical issues associated with vulnerable populations such as those at Letchworth Village are extremely important and relevant, this reference to the work of Koprowski is meant to convey his early work with a polio vaccine. For further information see: R. Kuschel, "The Necessity for Code of Ethics in Research," *Psihijatrija Danas*, 30(2–3)(1998), 247–74.

7. Albert Saban, http://www.nndb.com/people/180/000115832/.

8. Ibid.

9. Oshinsky, *Polio: An American Story*, 134.

10. "Salk versus Sabin: Great Polio Debate Revived," *The Southeast Missourian*, Oct 10, 1976.

11. Bonnie A. Maybury Okonek and Linda Morganstein, "Development of Polio Vaccines," *Access Excellence Classic Collection*, http://www.accessexcellence.org/AE/AEC/CC/polio.php.

12. Peter Cummings, "Salk and Sabin," *Brass Tacks*, March 2, 1963.

13. In the year 2000, the Centers for Disease Control (CDC) "endorsed a full return to the Salk vaccine in the United States." Oshinsky, *Polio: An American Story*, 279.

14. For more information, see http://www.salk.edu/.

15. In a document compiled at the March of Dimes Archives titled "March of Dimes Support to Tuskegee Institute, Annual Report Data, 1939 to 1967," archivist David Rose notes: "There are eight files of correspondence and reports on the HeLa Cell project, but while there are some accounting reports of budgets for Tuskegee staff, supplies, etc., there is no consistent report of year-by-year or grand totals relating to this project." In a letter from Henry Kumm to Basil O'Connor, September 15, 1955, March of Dimes Archives, Kumm notes that as of January 28, 1955, the NFIP had provided grants totaling $473,786.00.

16. Harry M. Weaver to Russell Brown, December 3, 1952.

17. Annual Report Data, 1939 to 1967.

18. March of Dimes, http://www.marchofdimes.com/.

19. Ibid.

20. *The Annual Report*, Carver Foundation, 1951–52, Tuskegee University notes that there was one scientist with a PhD in Foods and Nutrition, two in Poultry Husbandry, and three in Chemistry.

21. *Agenda for Annual Meeting Board of Trustees*, The Carver Research Foundation, Friday-Saturday, March 18–19, 1983.

22. Henry Kumm to Thomas Rivers, October 24, 1956, March of Dimes Archives.

23. Ibid.

24. Basil O'Connor to Luther Foster, October 29, 1956, March of Dimes Archives.

25. Russell Brown to T. E. Boyd, June 1, 1955, March of Dimes Archives.

26. Scientific Products Division, American Hospital Supply Corporation to Russell Brown, July 13, 1955, and David Preston to Russell Brown, July 28, 1955, March of Dimes Archives.

27. Russell Brown to T. E. Boyd, October 1, 1954, March of Dimes Archives.

28. Henry Kumm to Basil O'Connor, September 15, 1955, March of Dimes Archives.

29. Dr. Timothy Turner is currently a professor in the Department of Biology at Tuskegee University and the Tuskegee University Center for Cancer Research & Center for Biomedical Research/RCMI.

30. Timothy Turner, "Development of the Polio Vaccine: A Historical Perspective of Tuskegee University's Role in Mass Production and Distribution of HeLa Cells," *The Journal of Health Care for the Poor and Underserved* 23, no. 4 (2012): 5–10. https://muse.jhu.edu/, accessed July 29, 2016.

31. Brown and Henderson, writing in their article "The Mass Production and Distribution of HeLa Cells at Tuskegee Institute, 1953–55" refer to Henrietta Lacks as the progenitor of the cell cultures designated HeLa. They note: "the code name HeLa, designating the cell strain, was derived from the first two letters of Henrietta Lacks's first and last names." This document was written in 1981 and by no means indicates that they were aware of that fact prior to or during the NFIP designated field trials of which Tuskegee University's Carver Foundation was a part.

32. Smith, *Patenting the Sun*, 359–67.

33. Cutter Industries of Berkeley, California, was one of the four laboratories that had not participated in the original field trials. Ibid., 363.

34. First identified by Ben Sweet and Maurice Hilleman in 1960, Simian Virus or SV40 is an abbreviation for Simian vacuolating virus 40. SV40 is a polyomavirus that is found in both monkeys and humans and is a DNA virus that has the potential to cause tumors in animals, but most often persists as a latent infection. The scientists found that between 10 percent to 30 percent of polio vaccines in the United States were contaminated with SV40. B. H. Sweet and M. R. Hilleman, "The Vacuolating Virus, S.V. 40," *Proceedings of the Society for Experimental Biology and Medicine*, November 1960, 105 (2): 420–27.

35. For more information, see: "SV40 and polio vaccines," www.cdc.gov.

36. "Animal Cell Culture," *The Carver Research Foundation Annual Report, 1955–56*, No. 5.

37. Ibid.

38. "Growth Requirements of Animal Cells in Tissue Culture," *The Carver Foundation Annual Report, 1957–58*, No. 7.

39. "Tissue Culture," *The Carver Foundation Annual Report, 1958–59*, No. 8.

40. Ibid.

41. "Tissue Culture: Mammalian Cell Repository," *The Carver Foundation Annual Report, 1959–60*, No. 9. The Carver Research Foundation still works to eradicate disease, especially cancer, through cell culture manipulation. The list of Cell Strains in the Experimental Cell Repository at Tuskegee Institute During 1955 to 1961 (appendix 5) was taken from an unpublished paper with similar title to a previous document. The paper titled "The Ubiquitous HeLa Cell: Historic Account of the Mass Production and Distribution of HeLa Cells and Prototype Animal Cell Repository at Tuskegee Institute" by Russell W. Brown, William F. Scherer, Linda P. Washington, and James Henderson was produced in response to a March of Dimes grant, no. 1–753, dated March 1, 1981.

42. In a test tube, culture dish, etc.; hence, outside a living body, under artificial

conditions; also *attrib.*, performed, obtained, or occurring in vitro. Oxford English Dictionary, "in vitro," *Oxford English Dictionary* (Oxford, UK: Oxford University Press, 2014).

43. For further information see: "1950s: Prescriptions and Polio," *The Pharmaceutical Century: Ten Decades of Drug Discovery*, www2.uah.es/farmamol/The Pharmaceutical Century/Ch4.html (accessed September 19, 2013).

44. This study, March of Dimes #1–753, was funded at $10,000 for the year April 1981–March 31, 1982. The final paper was published in the *Journal of the History of Medicine*, Vol. 38, October 1983: 415–31. Proposal submitted from the President's Office, Tuskegee Institute, February 1981. The NFIP did not require an end of project publication, since it was on a quarterly contract basis with Tuskegee University. All that was required was an administrative, quarterly report. Finally, the NFIP published national news reports at the end of the trial.

45. "Transportation of Human Cells Culture in vitro," William F. Scherer and Russell W. Brown, *Proceedings of the Society for Experimental Biology and Medicine*, Vol. 92, 1956, 82–84.

46. The paper was presented at Brooks Air Force Base, Texas in 1966.

47. Ibid.

48. Brown, et al, "The Ubiquitous HeLa Cell," 32. See footnote no. 337.

49. Mayberry, *History of the Caver Research Foundation*, ix.

50. Gary R. Kramer, *George Washington Carver: In His Own Words* (Columbia: University of Missouri Press, 1987), 102.

51. "History," *March of Dimes: Working Together for Stronger, Healthier Babies*, http://www.marchofdimes.com/mission/a-history-of-the-march-of-dimes.aspx (accessed November 20, 2013).

52. Ibid.

53. Particularly, the March of Dimes would do this through assistance to newborn intensive care units (NICUs) such as in hospitals of the Gulf Coast states in 2005 in the aftermath of Hurricane Katrina.

54. Charles Bynum to Linda S. Franck, June 21, 1963, March of Dimes Archives.

55. Gregg Mitman, "The Color of Money: Campaigning for Health in Black and White America," 2003, March of Dimes Archives.

56. Interview with Edith Powell, November 20, 2013.

57. *Annual Reports of the President*, Tuskegee University, 1978–79.

58. Allied Health consisted of Radiologic Technology, Occupational Therapy, Physical Therapy and Clinical Laboratory Science (Medical Technology).

59. "Message from the President," *Annual Report of the President, 1988*, Tuskegee University.

60. Ibid.

61. These events have been accredited to the cooperation of Dr. Eugene Dibble. For more information, see: Reverby, *Examining Tuskegee*, 158.

62. William J. Cooper Jr. and Thomas E. Terrill, *The American South: A History*, 3d ed., 2 vols. (Boston: McGraw Hill, 2002).

63. Alabama's Black Belt refers to the rich, black soils that are a part of the piedmont.

64. The Second Reconstruction is "the broad period from the end of World War II until the late 1960s, often referred to as the 'Second Reconstruction,' consisted of a grass-roots civil rights movement coupled with gradual but progressive

actions by the Presidents, the federal courts, and Congress to provide full political rights for African Americans and to begin to redress longstanding economic and social inequities." The civil rights movement and the Second Reconstruction, 1945–1968, *History, Art and Archives: United States House of Representatives*, http://history .house.gov/Exhibitions-and-Publications/BAIC/Historical-Essays/Keeping-the -Faith/Civil-Rights-Movement/, accessed August 10, 2016.

Epilogue

1. "UAB/Tuskegee/Morehouse Partnership," UAB Comprehensive Cancer Outreach, http://www3.ccc.uab.edu/index.php?option=com_content&view=article &id=141&Itemid=147, accessed November 20, 2013.

2. Brochure, Johntyle Robinson, "The Patient, The Project, The Partnership: Mass Production & Distribution of HeLa Cells at Tuskegee University" (Tuskegee, University: The Legacy Museum, January 18, 2012), 7.

3. USPHSSS or US Public Health Service Syphilis Study.

References

"Analyzing Ethnic Education Policy-Making in England and Wales." *Sheffield Online Papers in Social Research.* Accessed June 20, 2006. https://www.sheffield.ac.uk/polopoly_fs/1.71426!/file/race_article.pdf.

"Animal Cell Culture." *The Carver Research Foundation Annual Report, 1955–56,* No. 5. Tuskegee, AL: Tuskegee Institute, 1956.

Annual Report of the George Washington Carver Foundation and a Resume of the Period, 1940–1947. Tuskegee, AL: Tuskegee Institute, 1948.

Annual Report of the President. Tuskegee, AL: Tuskegee Institute Press, 1947.

Aubrey, Harold L. "African Americans and the Broader Legacy of Experience with the American Health Care Community: Parasites, Locusts, and Scavengers." In *The Search for the Legacy of the USPHS Syphilis Study at Tuskegee,* edited by Ralph V. Katz and Rueben C. Warren, 107–16. New York: Lexington Books, 2011.

Baghdady, Maddock J. "Marching to a Different Mission." *Stanford Social Innovation Review:* 60–65 (Spring 2008). 61–65.

Bankston, John. *Jonas Salk and the Polio Vaccine.* Bear, DE: Mitchell Lane Publishers, 2002.

Barkan, E. *The Retreat of Scientific Racism: Changing Concepts of Race in Britain and the United States Between the World Wars.* Cambridge, UK: Cambridge University Press, 1992.

Bergman, Jerry. "A Brief History of the Eugenics Movement." *Investigator.* May, 2000. 72–77.

Black, Edwin. *War Against the Weak: Eugenics and America's Campaign to Create a Master Race.* New York: Dialog Press, 2003.

"Black Hospital Movement in Alabama." *Encyclopedia of Alabama.* Accessed May 12, 2015. http://www.encyclopediaofalabama.org/article/h-2410#sthash.QvjHnQ1M.dpuf.

Blakeslee, Alton. *Polio Can Be Conquered.* Washington: Public Affairs Committee, Incorporated, 1949.

———. *Polio and the Salk Vaccine: What You Should Know About It.* New York: Gossett and Dunlap, 1956.

Bonner, Thomas Neville. *Iconoclast: Abraham Flexner and a Life in Learning.* Baltimore: Johns Hopkins University Press, 2002.

Bord, Jessica De. "Informed Consent." *Ethics in Medicine*. University of Washington School of Medicine, 2014. Accessed June 12, 2014. https://depts.washington.edu/bioethx/topics/consent.html.

Brown, Elizabeth. "The Career of Dr. John A. Kenney," *Campus Digest* (Tuskegee, AL), December 2, 1944.

Brown, Russel W. and William F. Scherer, et al., "Report: The Ubiquitous HeLa Cell: Historic Account of the Mass Production and Distribution of HeLa Cells and Prototype Animal Cell Repository at Tuskegee Institute," Grant No. 1–753, March of Dimes/Birth Defects Foundation, March 1, 1981.

Brunner, Edmund and Hsin Pao Yang. *Rural America and the Extension Service*. New York: Bureau of Publications, Teachers College, Columbia University, 1949.

Burchard, Peter Duncan. *George Washington Carver: For His Time and Ours*. Diamond, Missouri: United States Department of the Interior Printing, 2005.

Campbell, Thomas Monroe. *Movable School Goes to The Negro Farmer*. Tuskegee, AL: Tuskegee Institute Press, 1936.

Carroll, William R. and Merle E. Muhrer. "The Scientific Contributions of George Washington Carver." Unpublished report for National Park Service, 1962.

Cerami, Charles. *Benjamin Banneker: Surveyor, Astronomer, Publisher, Patriot*. New York: John Wiley & Sons, Inc., 2002.

Chandler, Dana R. "Tuskegee University." In *The New Encyclopedia of Southern Culture, Volume 17, Education*, edited by Clarence L. Mohr, 323–26. Chapel Hill: The University of North Carolina Press, 2011.

Chenault, John W. "Infantile Paralysis (Acute Anterior Poliomyelitis)." *Journal of the National Medical Association*. 33:221 (1941): 220–26.

The Chicago Manual of Style, Sixteenth Edition. Chicago: University of Chicago Press, 2010.

"The Civil Rights Movement and the Second Reconstruction, 1945–1968," *History, Art and Archives: United States House of Representatives*, Accessed August 10, 2016. http://history.house.gov/Exhibitions-and-Publications/BAIC/Historical-Essays/Keeping-the-Faith/Civil-Rights-Movement/.

Cobbs v. Grant (8 Cal. 3d 229) 1972. *Law and Bioethics*. Accessed May 18, 2014. http://www.lawandbioethics.com/demo/Main/LegalResources/C5/Cobbs.htm.

Collins, David. *Practical Rules for the Management and Medical Treatment of Negro Slaves in the Sugar Colonies*. London: J. Barfield, 1811.

Cooper, William J. Jr. and Thomas E. Terrill. 2002. *The American South: A History*, 3d ed., 2 vols. Boston: McGraw Hill, 2002.

"County Health Departments." *Alabama Public Health*. Accessed February 25, 2016. http://www.adph.org/administration/Default.asp?id=505.

Crosby, E. W. "The Roots of Black Agricultural Extension Work." *Historian*, 39 (2009): 228–47.

Cummings, Peter. "Salk and Sabin," *Brass Tacks*, (Boston, MA), March 2, 1963.

Cushing, Harvey. *The Life of Sir William Osler*. Oxford, UK: Clarendon Press, 1925.

The C. V. Roman Public Health Meeting. Tuskegee, AL: Tuskegee Institute. April 1949.

Daniel, Peter. "Black Power in the 1920s: The Case of the Tuskegee Veteran's Hospital." *Journal of Southern History* 36 (August 1970): 368–88.

Daniel, T. M. and F. C. Robbins. "A History of Poliomyelitis." *Polio* (1997): 5–22.

Davis, Charles G. "Historical Address." In *Addresses Delivered at the Massachusetts*

Agricultural College, June 21st, 1887, on the 25th Anniversary of the Passage of the Morrill Land Grant Act. Amherst, Mass: J. E. Williams, 1887.

Denton, Virginia Lantz. *Booker T. Washington and the Adult Education Movement*. Gainesville: University Press of Florida, 1993.

Dikotter, Frank. "Race Culture: Recent Perspectives on the History of Eugenics." *The American Historical Review* 103 (April, 1998): 2.

Dorsette, Cornelius Nathaniel. *Encyclopedia of Alabama*. Accessed May 11, 2015. http://www.encyclopediaofalabama.org/article/h-3282.

"Dr. John A. Kenney Leaves Tuskegee." *Journal of the National Medical Association* 36.6 (1944): 199–200.

Du Bois, W. E. B. *Black Folk, Then and Now: An Essay in the History and Sociology of the Negro Race*. New York: H. Holt and Company, 1939.

"Editorial." *The Southern Workman*. April, 1921.

Edwards, Ethel. *Carver of Tuskegee*. Tuskegee, Alabama: Privately Published, 1971.

Eiseman, Elisa. and Susanne B. Haga. *Handbook of Human Tissue Sources: A National Resource of Human Tissue Samples*. Santa Monica, CA: Rand Corporation, 1999.

Ellingson, Terry Jay. *The Myth of the Noble Savage*. Oakland: University of California Press, 2001.

Erickson, Paul A. and Liam D. Murphy. "Scientific racism: Improper or incorrect science that actively or passively supports racism." *A History of Anthropological Theory*. Toronto: UTP Higher Education, 2008.

"Events 1901–1970." *Liberia*. Alabama Public Television. Accessed December 12, 2012. http://www.pbs.org/wgbh/globalconnections/liberia/timeline/time3.html.

Ferguson, George O. *The Psychology of the Negro*. Westport, CT: Negro Universities Press, 1916.

Fett, Sharla. *Working Cures: Healing, Health, and Power on Southern Slave Plantations*. Chapel Hill: University of North Carolina Press, 2002.

"The First Female Physician in Alabama." *Birmingham Medical News*. Accessed May 12, 2015. http://www.birminghammedicalnews.com/news.php?viewStory=1530.

Fisher, John E. *The John F. Slater Fund: A Nineteenth Century Affirmative Action for Negro Education*. New York: University Press of America, 1896.

Fosdick, Raymond Blaine. *Adventures in Giving: The Story of the General Education Board*. New York: Harper and Row, 1962.

Four Eulogies. White Plains, NY: The Nation Foundation-March of Dimes, 1972.

Francis, Thomas, et al. *Evaluation of the 1954 Field Trial of Poliomyelitis Vaccine: Final Report*. Ann Arbor, MI: Edwards Brothers, Inc., 1957.

Gamble, Vanessa Northington. *Making a Place for Ourselves: The Black Hospital Movement, 1920–1945*. New York: Oxford University Press, 1995.

"A Good Work Goes Forward." *Birmingham News*. February 5, 1949.

Garrett, Laurie. *Betrayal of Trust: The Collapse of Global Public Health*. New York: Hyperion, 2011.

George Washington Carver Foundation Board of Directors, *Minutes of the Annual Meeting*. February 10, 1953.

Gilliam, Charles P. "A Short History of the National Grange of the Order of Patrons of Husbandry." *Cannongrange*. Accessed July 28, 2016. http://www.oocities.org/cannongrange/cannon_nationalhistory.html.

Gobineau, Arthur de. *An Essay on the Inequality of the Human Races*. New York: G. P. Putnam and Sons, 1915.

Goode, Sarah. "Inventors." *The Black Inventor On-Line Museum*, 2011.

Gould, Stephen J. "American Polygeny and Craniometry Before Darwin." *The "Racial" Economy of Science: Toward a Democratic Future*, edited by Sandra Harding, 84–115. Bloomington: Indiana University Press, 1993.

Graham, Shirley and George D. Lipscomb. *Dr. George Washington Carver, Scientist*. New York: Simon & Schuster, Inc., 1972.

"Growth Requirements of Animal Cells in Tissue Culture." *The Carver Foundation Annual Report, 1957–58*, No. 7.

Hand, Wayland D. *Popular Beliefs and Superstitions from North Carolina*. vols. 6 and 7 (1961, 1964).

Harlan, Louis R. *The Booker T. Washington Papers*, Vol. 3. Urbana: University of Illinois Press, 1974.

Hayes, Helen. *My Life in Three Acts*. San Diego: Harcourt Brace Jovanovich, 1990.

Henry, Ava and Michael Williams. *Black Scientists and Inventors Book One*. London: BIS Enterprises Ltd., 2002.

Hicks, Cheryl D. *Talk with You Like a Woman: African American Women, Justice, and Reform in New York, 1890–1925*. Chapel Hill: University of North Carolina Press, 2010.

Higgins, A. C. "Scientific Racism: A review of *The Science and Politics of Racial Research* by William H. Tucker." *Mathematicians of the African Diaspora*. Chicago: University of Illinois Press, 1994.

"Hilary Koprowski, Who Developed First Live-Virus Polio Vaccine, Dies at 96." *New York Times*. April 20, 2013.

Hild, Matthew. "Farmer's Alliance." *New Georgia Encyclopedia*. Acccessed July 28, 2016. http://www.georgiaencyclopedia.org/articles/history-archaeology/farmers -alliance.

Hines, Darlene Clark. *Black Women in White: Racial Conflict and Cooperation in the Nursing Profession, 1890–1950*. Bloomington: Indiana University Press, 1989.

"History." *American Red Cross*. Accessed April 11, 2017. http://www.redcross.org/ about-us/who-we-are/history.

"History." *March of Dimes: Working Together for Stronger, Healthier Babies*. Accessed November 20, 2013. http://www.marchofdimes.com/mission/a-history-of-the -march-of-dimes.aspx.

Holsey, Albon L. *Booker T. Washington's Own Story of His Life and Work*. Tuskegee, AL: Booker T. Washington, 1901.

Holt, Rackham. *George Washington Carver, An American Biography*. Garden City, NY: Doubleday and Co., 1943.

Imes, G. Lake. *The Philosophies of Booker T. Washington*. Tuskegee, AL: Tuskegee Institute Press, 1941.

The Infantile Paralysis Fight at Tuskegee. New York: National Foundation for Infantile Paralysis, 1948.

"In Memoriam." *American Historical Association Perspectives*. October 2007, 45:7.

"In the 1930s, Scientists Measured Black College Students to Define the 'Negro Race.'" *BuzzFeed News*. Accessed March 17, 2016. http://www.buzzfeed.com/ danvergano/tuskegee-student-measurements.

"Intertwined Destinies." *Montgomery Advertiser*. April 6, 1956.

Isaac, Joel. *Working Knowledge: Making the Human Sciences from Parsons to Kuhn.* Cambridge, MA: Harvard University Press, 2012.

Jackson Jr., John P. and Nadine M. Weidman. *Race, Racism, and Science: Social Impact and Interaction.* Santa Barbara, CA: ABC-CLIO, Inc., 2004.

"Jim Crow Laws (Examples)." Martin Luther King Jr National Historic Site Interpretive Staff. Accessed January 5, 1998. http://www.nps.gove/malu/documents/jim_crow_laws.htm.

"John A. Andrew Memorial Hospital." *Tuskegee Student,* Vol. 25, No. 5 (1913), 4.

Jones, Gwyn E. and Chris Garforth, "The history, development, and future of agricultural extension." Accessed December 15, 2015. http://www.fao.org/docrep/w5830e/w5830e03.htm.

Jones, James. *Bad Blood: The Tuskegee Syphilis Experiment.* New York: The Free Press, 1981.

Kaplan, Mary. *The Tuskegee Veterans Hospital and Its Black Physicians: The Early Years.* Jefferson, NC: McFarland and Company, Inc., 2016.

Karenga, Maulana. *Introduction to Black Studies,* 3rd edition. Timbuktu, Mali: University of Sankore Press, 2002.

Katz, J. *The Silent World of Doctor and Patient.* Baltimore: Johns Hopkins University Press, 2002.

Kenny, Elizabeth. *The Kenny Concept of Infantile Paralysis, and Its Treatment.* St. Paul, MN: Bruce Publishing Co., 1943.

Koseluk, Gregory. *Eddie Cantor: A Life in Show Business.* Jefferson, NC: McFarland & Co., 1995.

Kramer, Gary R. *George Washington Carver: In His Own Words.* Columbia: University of Missouri Press, 1987.

Kuper, Adam and Jessica Kuper, eds., "Racism." *The Social Science Encyclopedia.* 1996.

Kuschel, R. "The Necessity for Code of Ethics in Research." *Psihijatrija Danas,* 30(2–3) (1998): 247–74.

Lapouge, Georges Vacher de and C. Clossen. "Old and New Aspects of the Aryan Question." *The American Journal of Sociology* 5 (3): 329–46.

Leclerc, Georges-Louis. *Comte de Buffon, Natural History, General and Particular.* Translated by William Smellie. Bristol, UK: Thoemmes Press, 2000.

Lippman, Theo, Jr. *The Squire of Warm Springs: F.D.R. in Georgia, 1924–1945.* Chicago: Playboy, 1977.

Lombardo, Paul A. "Anthropometry, Race, and Eugenic Research: Measurements of Growing Negro Children at the Tuskegee Institute, 1932–1944." In *The Uses of Humans in Experiment: Perspectives from the 17th to the 20th Century,* edited by Erika Dyck and Larry, 215–39. Stewart. Boston: Brill Rodopi, 2016.

Lombardo, Paul A. and Gregory M. Dorr. 2006 "Eugenics, Medical Education, and the Public Health Service: Another Perspective on the Tuskegee Syphilis Experiment." *Bulletin of the History of Medicine* 80(2): 291–316.

Long, Carolyn Morrow. *Spiritual Merchants: Religion, Magic and Commerce.* Knoxville: University of Tennessee Press, 2001.

Ludden, Forrest E. *The History of Public Health in Alabama, 1941–1968.* Montgomery: Alabama Department of Public Health, 1970.

Marshall, Gloria A. "Racial Classifications Popular and Scientific." *The "Racial" Economy of Science: Toward a Democratic Future,* edited by Sandra Harding, 116–27. Bloomington: Indiana University Press, 1993.

Madigan, Michael and John Martinko, eds. *Brock Biology of Microorganisms*. Cranbury, NJ: Prentice Hall, 2005.

Matthews, Holly. "Doctors and Root Doctors: Patients Who Use Both," in James Kirkland and others, eds., *Herbal and Magical Medicine: Traditional Healing Today*: 71–93. Durham, NC: Duke University Press, 1992.

Mawdsley, Stephen E. " 'Dancing on Eggs': Charles H. Bynum, Racial Politics, and the National Foundation for Infantile Paralysis, 1938–1954." *Bulletin of the History of Medicine*. 84, 2 (Summer 2010): 217–47.

Mayberry, B. D. *A Century of Agriculture in the 1890 Land-Grant Institutions and Tuskegee University—1890–1990*. New York: Vintage Press, 1991.

———. *The History of the Carver Research Foundation of Tuskegee University*. Tuskegee, AL: Tuskegee University Press, 2003.

———. *Role of Tuskegee University in the Origin, Growth and Development of the Negro Cooperative Extension System, 1881–1990*. Montgomery, AL: Brown Printing Co., 1989.

McMurray, Linda O. *George Washington Carver: Scientist and Symbol*. Oxford, UK: Oxford University Press, 1981.

Mehetre, S. S. and A. R. Aher. "Embryo rescue: A tool to overcome incompatible interspecific hybridization in *Gossypium* Linn, a review," *Indian Journal of Biotechnology* 3: 29–36 (2004).

Miller, Linda Kenney. *Beacon on the Hill*. Dallas, TX: Harper House Publishers, 2008.

———. *The Negro in Medicine*. Marietta, GA: Harper House Publishers, 2008.

Montagu, M. F. Ashley. *Man's Most Dangerous Myth: The Fallacy of Race*. New York: Columbia University Press, 1942.

Moore, W. 2013. "Red Pill Hangovers, Covert Racism, and the Sociological Machine." *American Sociological Association* 42 (2013):529–32.

Morais, Herbert. *The History of the Afro-American in Medicine*. Cornwells Heights, PA: The Publishing Agency, Inc., 1976.

Moton, Robert R. *Annals of the Academy of Political and Social Science* 140:257–263; n. 1928.

"1950s: Prescriptions and Polio." *The Pharmaceutical Century: Ten Decades of Drug Discovery*. Accessed September 19, 2013. www2.uah.es/farmamol/The Pharmaceutical Century/Ch4.html.

"Nobel Lectures." *Physiology or Medicine 1942–1962*. Amsterdam, Elsevier Publishing CO., 1964.

Nordenberg, Chancellor Mark A. *Defeat of an Enemy*. Pittsburgh: University of Pittsburgh Press, 2015.

Norrell, Robert. *Up from History: The Life of Booker T. Washington*. New York: Belknap Press, 2011.

OHA 316 Steggerda Collection. Otis Historical Archives. *National Museum of Health and Medicine*. Accessed March 17, 2016. http://www.medicalmuseum.mil/assets/documents/collections/archives/2014/OHA%20316%20Steggerda%20Collection.pdf.

Okonek, Bonnie A. Maybury and Linda Morganstein. "Development of Polio Vaccines." *Access Excellence Classic Collection*. Accessed March 17, 2015. http://www.accessexcellence.org/AE/AEC/CC/polio.php.

"Opening Doors: Contemporary African American Academic Surgeons." *US Na-*

tional Library of Medicine. Accessed August 10, 2016. https://www.nlm.nih.gov/exhibition/aframsurgeons/history.html.

Oshinsky, David M. *Polio: An American Story.* Oxford, UK: Oxford University Press, 2005.

Paul, John R. *A History of Poliomyelitis.* New Haven: Yale University Press, 1971.

Peakman, Mark and Diego Vergani. *Basic and Clinical Immunology, 2nd Edition.* London: Churchill Livingstone, 2009.

Peyton, Thomas Roy. *Quest for Dignity: An Autobiography of a Negro Doctor.* Los Angeles: Publishers Western, 1963.

Pina, A. S., A. Hussain, and A. C. Roque. "An historical overview of drug discovery." *Methods of Molecular Biology* 572 (2009): 3–12.

Poindexter, Hildrus A. *My World of Reality.* Detroit, MI: Balamp Publishing Co., 1973.

"Poliomyelitis Vaccine Types 1, 2, and 3." *Recommendations of Vaccine Advisory Committee,* 300–305. White Plains, NY: National Foundation for Infantile Paralysis, 1954.

Porter, Theodore M. and Dorothy Ross, eds. *The Cambridge History of Science: The Modern Social Sciences.* Cambridge, UK: Cambridge University Press, 2003.

Powell, Edith and John F. Hume. *A Black Oasis: Tuskegee Institute's Fight Against Infantile Paralysis, 1941–1975.* Montgomery, AL: McQuick Printing, 2008.

"Protecting and Promoting Your Health." *US Food and Drug Administration.* Accessed on March 7, 2016. http://www.fda.gov/EmergencyPreparedness/Counterterrorism/MedicalCountermeasures/ucm410308.htm.

Quinn, Sandra Course and Stephen B. Thomas. "The National Negro Health Week, 1915 to 1951: A Descriptive Account." *Minority Health Today,* 2 (3), 2001:44.

"Race, theories of." *Routledge Encyclopedia of Philosophy: Questions to Sociobiology.* New York: Routledge, 1998.

Railsback, Bruce. *What Is Science.* Accessed July 27, 2016. http://www.gly.uga.edu/railsback/1122science2.html.

Rasmussen, W. D. *Taking the University to the People: Seventy-Five Years of Cooperative Extension.* Ames: Iowa State University, 1989.

Reverby, Susan. *Examining Tuskegee: The Infamous Syphilis Study and Its Legacy.* Chapel Hill: University of North Carolina Press, 2009.

———. *Tuskegee's Truths: Rethinking the Tuskegee Syphilis Study.* Chapel Hill: University of North Carolina Press, 2000.

Rice, Mitchell F. and Woodrow Jones Jr. *Public Policy and the Black Hospital.* Westport, CT: Greenwood Press, 1994.

Ripley, William Z. *The Races of Europe: A Sociological Study.* Lowell Institute Lectures. London: K. Paul Trench, Trubner & Co., Ltd., 1913.

Robert Russa Moton of Hampton and Tuskegee. Edited by William Hardin Hughes and Frederick D. Patterson. Chapel Hill: University of North Carolina Press, 1956.

Robinson, Jontyle. "The Patient, The Project, The Partnership: Mass Production & Distribution of HeLa Cells at Tuskegee University" Tuskegee, AL: The Legacy Museum, 2012.

Rodgers, Samuel. "Kansas City General Hospital No. 2." *The Journal of the National Medical Association.* September 1, 1962: 525–44.

Rogers, Naomi. "Race and the Politics of Polio: Warm Springs, Tuskegee, and the March of Dimes." *American Journal of Public Health*. May 2007, 97(5): 784–95.

Rose, David. *Friends and Partners: The Legacy of Franklin D. Roosevelt and Basil O'Connor in the History of Polio*. Boston: Academic Press, 2016.

——. *Images of America: March of Dimes*. Charleston, SC: Arcadia Publishing, 2003.

Rosenberg, Charles E. *No Other Gods: On Science and American Social Thought*. Baltimore: Johns Hopkins University Press, 1997.

"Salk versus Sabin: Great Polio Debate Revived." *The Southeast Missourian*. October 10, 1976.

Sass, E. J. G. Gottfried and A. Sore. *Polio's Legacy: An Oral History*. Washington, DC: University Press of America, 1996.

Scott, Roy Vernon. *The Reluctant Farmer: The Rise of Agricultural Extension to 1914*. Urbana: University of Illinois Press, 1971.

Seavey, Nina, dir. *A Paralyzing Fear: The Story of Polio in America*. 1998; Burbank, CA: Public Broadcasting System (PBS), 1998. DVD.

Seham, Max. *Blacks and American Medical Care*. Minneapolis: University of Minnesota Press, 1973.

Selected Speeches of Booker T. Washington. Edited by E. Davidson Washington. Garden City, New York: Doubleday, Doran and Company, Inc., 1932.

"Sesquicentennial." *The Tuskegee News*. March 15, 1984.

Shors, Teri. *Understanding Viruses*. Burlington, MA: Jones and Bartlett Publishers, 2008.

Skloot, Rebecca. *The Immortal Life of Henrietta Lacks*. New York: Crown Publishing Group, 2010.

Smith, James W. "The Contributions of Black Americans to Agricultural Extension and Research." Accessed December 8, 2015. http://ageconsearch.umn.edu/bitstream/17424/1/ar840003.pdf.

Smith, Jane S. *Patenting the Sun: Polio and the Salk Vaccine, the Dramatic Story Behind One of the Greatest Achievements of Modern Science*. New York: William Morrow and Company, Inc., 1990.

Smith, Jean Edward. *FDR*. New York: Random House, 2008.

Smith, Susan L. "Neither Victim nor Villain." *Journal of Women's History*. 8 (1) (1996): 95–113.

——. *Sick and Tired of Being Sick and Tired Black Women's Health Activism in America, 1890–1950*. Philadelphia: University of Pennsylvania Press, 1995.

Smith, W. B. *The Color Line*. New York: Negro Universities Press, 1969.

Sullivan, Louis W. "The Education of Black Health Professionals," *Phylon* (1960–), Vol. 38, No. 2 (1977): 183.

Summerville, James. 2002. *Educating Black Doctors: A History of Meharry Medical College*. Tuscaloosa: University of Alabama Press, 2002.

Sweet, B. H. and M. R. Hilleman. "The Vacuolating Virus, S.V. 40." *Proceedings of the Society for Experimental Biology and Medicine*, November 1960, 105 (2): 420–27.

Taylor, Quintard. "An Online Reference Guide to African American History." *BlackPast*. Accessed December 14, 2012. www.blackpast.org/?q=aah/national-medical-association-1895.

Thomas, Alexander and Samuel Sillen. *Racism and Psychiatry* (New York: Brunner/Mazel, Inc., 1972).

Tindall, George B. *The Emergence of the New South, 1913–1945*. Baton Rouge: Louisiana State University Press, 1967.

"Tissue Culture: Mammalian Cell Repository." *The Carver Foundation Annual Report, 1959–60*, No. 9.

"Tissue Culture." *The Carver Foundation Annual Report, 1958–59*, No. 8.

Title 7. US Code, 304.

Title 7. US Code, 307.

Title 7. US Code, 343.

"Transportation of Human Cells Culture in vitro." William F. Scherer and Russell W. Brown, *Proceedings of the Society for Experimental Biology and Medicine*, Vol. 92, (1956): 82–84.

Troan, John. "How 'fooling around with polio thing led to a medical miracle." *Pittsburgh Tribune-Review*. April 3, 2005.

Turner, Timothy. "Development of the Polio Vaccine: A Historical Perspective of Tuskegee University's Role in Mass Production and Distribution of HeLa Cells." *The Journal of Health Care for the Poor and Underserved* 23, no. 4 (2012): 5–10. Accessed July 29, 2016. https://muse.jhu.edu/.

The Tuskegee Alumni Bulletin. 1920–1929.

Tuskegee Institute Annual Report of the President, 1955–1956.

The Tuskegee University Bulletin Courses and Programs: 1881–1882.

The Tuskegee University Bulletin Courses and Programs: 2004–2006.

"Tuskegee VA Medical Center Celebrates 85 Years of Service." *Central Alabama Veterans Health Care System*. Accessed December 13, 2012. http://www.centralalabama.va.gov/Press_Release.asp.

"Tuskegee Veterans Administration Hospital." *Alabama Travel*. Accessed December 13, 2012. http://www.alabama.travel/things-to-do/attractions/tuskegee_veterans_administration-hospital.

"UAB/Tuskegee/Morehouse Partnership," *UAB Comprehensive Cancer Outreach*. Accessed November 20, 2013. http://www3.ccc.uab.edu/index.php?option=com_content&view=article&id=141&Itemid=147.

Ward, Thomas J. Jr. *Black Physicians in the Jim Crow South*. Fayetteville: University of Arkansas Press, 2003.

Warren, Wini. *Black Women Scientists in the United States*. Bloomington: Indiana University Press, 2000.

Washington, Booker T. "The Negro Doctor in the South." *The Independent*. 1907.

———. *Southern Workman*, Vol. 10, No. 9.

———. *Up from Slavery*. New York: Doubleday, Page and Co., 1901.

———. *Working with the Hands*. New York: Doubleday, Page & Co., 1904.

Washington, Booker T, with the collaboration of Robert E. Park. *The Man Farthest Down: A Record of Observation and Study in Europe*. Garden City, NY: Doubleday, Page and Co., 1912.

Weiss, Ellen. *Robert R. Taylor and Tuskegee: An African American Architect Designs for Booker T. Washington*. Montgomery, AL: New South Books, 2012.

Wilder, Marshall P. *Address Delivered Before the Norfolk Agricultural Society, on the Occasion of its First Annual Exhibition, at Dedham*. Boston: The Society, 1849.

Wilson, Edward O. *Consilience: The Unity of Knowledge*. New York: Random House, 1999.

Woloch, Nancy. *Women and the American Experience.* 5th ed. New York: McGraw Hill, 2011.

"Women's Roles in the 1950s." *American Decades.* Vol. 6. 2001. Gale Group. Accessed July 16, 2008. http://find.galegroup.com.

Work, Monroe N. 1913–1943. *The Negro Year Book.* Tuskegee, AL: Tuskegee.

Wrenshall, C. Lewis. "The American Peanut Industry." *Economic Botany,* III (April–June 1949): 168.

Zabawa, Robert. "Tuskegee Institute Movable School." *Encyclopedia of Alabama.* Accessed January 26, 2016. http://www.encyclopediaofalabama.org/article/h -1870#sthash.PInnBgF9.dpuf.

Index